T0294415

PROJECT
UN
THINK
ABLE

PROJECT UN THINK ABLE

A DOCTOR'S GAMBLE TO SAVE MILLIONS OF LIVES

DR. DEREK YACH

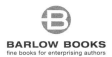

BARLOW BOOKS
fine books for enterprising authors

Library and Archives Canada Cataloguing in Publication data available upon request.

ISBN 978-1-988025-28-5 (hardcover)
ISBN 978-1-988025-30-8 (ebook)

Printed in Canada

To Order in Canada:
 Georgetown Publications
 34 Armstrong Avenue, Georgetown, ON L7G 4R9

To Order in the U.S.A.:
 Midpoint Book Sales & Distribution
 27 West 20th Street, Suite 1102, New York, NY 10011

Publisher   **Sarah Scott**
Book producer   **Tracy Bordian/At Large Editorial Services**
Cover design   **Paul Hodgson**
Interior design and page layout   **Kyle Gell**
Copy editor   **Eleanor Gasparik**
Proofreader   **Wendy Thomas**
Indexing   **Wendy Thomas**
Marketing and publicity   **Jared Kuritz/Strategies**

For more information, visit **www.barlowbooks.com**

Barlow Book Publishing Inc.
96 Elm Avenue, Toronto, ON
Canada M4W 1P2

**BARLOW
BOOKS**

■

To my wife, Yasmin, for almost four decades of intellectual and emotional support, helpful critique, and loving guidance in a world of tough choices.

To my son, Julian, to help you understand what I have tried to achieve through my work and time away from you.

To the billion-plus smokers for whom I lacked empathy and failed for the longest time to include in the battle — mea culpa.

■

CONTENTS

PROLOGUE

September 2015, John F. Kennedy International Airport: I am on an evening flight from New York to Geneva, a journey I have made often over the last decade but never for this purpose. From my seat in business class, from behind my glasses, I surreptitiously glance up to scrutinize the faces of the passengers around me. Do I know them from somewhere? Do they know me? I recognize no one. Relief floods through my body, and I sink further into the comfortable seat, headphones on, hoping to lose myself in a movie. But I can't concentrate. My mind is racing ahead to arrival at Geneva Airport, which is like a second home for people I used to work with as they fly to and from meetings around the world.

Just like I am.

Only a few years ago, that airport was my second home, too, as part of a high-flying job I had at the World Health Organization. What if I run into an old friend or former colleague when I get there? I have no idea what I will say. Silently, I test out different responses to see how they would go over.

"I'm here to do some touring."

No. I'm hardly a tourist, having lived here for nearly ten years.

Or "There's a swimming competition I'm going to on Lake Geneva. You remember that I love to swim?"

I may be an avid swimmer but travelling to Switzerland in the fall to participate in a competition somehow beggars belief.

Or, more simply, "I am visiting old friends."

I reject that one, too. The friends my wife Yasmin and I had in the region—doctors, scientists, and peers—are the very ones I would be making excuses to, because I can't tell them the truth in the first place.

The fact is, I am going to a meeting at Philip Morris International Inc.

There, I've said it to myself. There is no getting around it. If it was anyone else, that might sound reasonable or at least acceptable; but for me, it encompasses the impossible—the unthinkable. I, an epidemiologist and public health expert, the first-ever director of the World Health Organization's Tobacco Free Initiative, and an architect of the international treaty known as the Framework Convention on Tobacco

Control—conceived to protect present and future genera-tions from the devastating health, social, environmental, and economic consequences of tobacco consumption and exposure to its deadly smoke—am en route to the Lausanne headquarters of the second-largest cigarette manufacturer in the world.

I have spent my entire adult life fighting tobacco companies and the lies they have told. I helped enact a set of universal standards and provisions that include rules to govern the production, sale, distribution, advertising, and taxation of tobacco products, which in turn have led to a 2.5 per cent reduction in global smoking rates. That may not sound like much, but when you consider that around the world about 1.1 billion people, or one in three adults, smoke, that per-centage is huge. And yet, here I am, on my way to a date with Philip Morris International (PMI) chief executive officer André Calantzopoulos.

Is it any wonder I'm nervous? If I do encounter someone I know at the airport, I shall have to be purposefully vague about the visit and hope that I am not pressed further. Or I will pull up the collar of my woollen trench coat and duck my head to hide my face. Or just hurry by, a scurrying figure in rumpled clothes he has slept in on the plane.

Don't panic. Breathe. Pace yourself. It's just a meeting.

Truth be told, I still can't quite believe I'm here, high above the Atlantic, eating a meal, reclining my seat, putting on an eye mask to sleep for a few hours as the plane hurtles me toward a place of business I have spent the whole of my professional life trying to destroy.

The statistics run through my mind in an endless loop: cigarettes kill about seven million people a year around the world right now and are projected to kill up to one billion in this century.[1] Tobacco use means disease and death, period. And yet here I am, travelling to a factory in the business of death, one of the five big players in an industry that for years bribed government officials and academics to take their side; an industry that prevaricated, obfuscated, and outright lied when presented with incontrovertible facts, with scientific research and statistics about the link between cigarettes and cancer; an industry that balked every step of the way as we worked toward the signing of the international treaty, even setting paid spies in our midst.

I know I risk censure and ostracism from my scientific colleagues who, given Big Tobacco's dismal track record, dismiss any claims by the companies that they're trying to do the right thing. For much of the public health community, the only way to diminish tobacco's influence is through education, hardline legislation, higher excise taxes, help for addicts to go cold turkey, or, in the best and most unlikely scenario of all, shutting down the companies.

They will say I have been bought.

They will say I am doing the unthinkable.

To the first charge, I can respond with a definitive "no." As to the second, they are absolutely right. Ever since I was a child, I've had a stubborn streak, always insisting on look-ing at every side of every problem, turning it upside down and inside out. And when a new, previously unthinkable angle comes up that has the potential to change the way we approach that problem, something in me needs to see it through to the end, no matter the price I may have to pay. I shall have to be strong, stronger than I have had to be before.

Maybe I'm naive, but I like to believe that people, and even whole industries, can change their opinions and approach. Or at the very least, they can shift their priorities, which may be change enough in itself. Maybe I just like to keep an open mind. Growing up in South Africa under apartheid, I learned early to have faith that the racist, repressive system of gov-ernment would change. It had to. Why *not* Philip Morris?

On the plane, I carry no notes because I very deliberately didn't write anything down. I didn't want to take a chance that anyone would see them. Instead, I mentally review the conditions and questions I have, the studies and statistics I have been poring over—I want to be able to call upon them without a moment's hesitation. In one of his books, Henry Kissinger wrote that whenever he sees people in meetings or other settings, he knows that even if he simply smiles and says "hello," that will lead to something else and he has to be prepared to handle what comes next, and next, and next.

I know I'm on my way to a meeting that could change the course of my life and the future of people's health. So, I will channel Henry Kissinger. I will force myself to be calm, and my mantra shall be "Listen, respond, be prepared for what comes, and do not judge."

The pilot announces our descent into Geneva. There is no going back.

A new wave of sudden panic.

What if—oh, my God—what if the driver from Philip Morris is waiting for me with a sign that says "PMI—Derek Yach"?

For a moment, the image is my nightmare come to life. I'd have nowhere to hide. Maybe people I know have already seen the sign (if it exists) and have charged, tried, and convicted me with my having no say in the matter.

Don't be silly, I chide myself. Like it or not, hide it or not, I am about to do the unthinkable—again. The plane taxis to a standstill at the gate. I stand up to shrug on my coat.

BEGINNINGS

Cape Town, South Africa: I am four years old, and plunged suddenly into water. There is no time to be scared. I try to keep my breathing deep and even, with my legs pedalling furiously in an effort to keep my head up and to stay afloat.

I can hear shouting.

"Come on, Derek!"

"Arms! Use your arms!"

"Go! Go!"

In my head, I can hear my father, an Olympic swimmer in his youth and one of the country's top freestylers, instructing me in a quiet voice that betrays no emotion. "Stay calm," he says. "Think of what you need to do and then do it."

Though I feel adrift in the middle of an ocean, I'm actually in my maternal grandfather's pool in the garden of his Cape Town home. Shaped like an elongated heart, it has a border of black-painted wood that absorbs the heat from the South African sun, making it hot and hard to stand at the edge in bare feet. Until this moment, I have only ever ventured into the shallow end; now I have been picked up, thrown into the deep end, and told to swim. There is no life jacket, no water wings to help keep me afloat, no adult to gently cradle my torso. Swim, or sink. To my young mind, it's that stark a choice, even though I know that someone will jump in to help if I need it. I'm determined to do it on my own. I can just make out the lush green grass beyond the pool's edge. It looks unreal, like streaks of paint. Palm trees stand sentinel over the scene, impervious and still, and too far away.

And so, I perform an inelegant dog paddle with my head held aloft, moving toward a long pole a teacher named Mrs. Mack proffers over the pool's edge. My effort lasts no more than thirty seconds, but it instills in me the knowledge not that I can do anything but, rather, that I should not be scared to try. When I am hauled out, dripping, shivering, and proud, that knowledge settles in my gut. Be brave. Be tough. Take risks and, most of all, don't be afraid to fail.

As I'm wrapped in a towel, I hear my father say: "Well done. Next time will be even better."

My father, Solm, or "Solly" to his friends, was a man who dove in and saw a swim through to the end, no matter how hard the slog or how rough the water got. I wanted to be like him.

◼

Growing up in Cape Town in the late 1950s and '60s, the second of my parents' four children (and the oldest of their three sons), my grandparents' experiences and values made as much of an imprint on me as did those of my own parents. I heard the stories. My father told me of how his own father, Aaron Yach, an observant Jew who landed in South Africa in the 1920s after fleeing pogroms in Lithuania a few years earlier, went against all the tenets he believed in when he asked the rabbi to grant his son special dispensation from attending synagogue and resting on the Sabbath because swim meets were invariably held on that day. This would have been unthinkable back in the old country, where tradition ruled, but my grandfather, who spoke mainly Yiddish until the day he died, understood the importance of adapting and occasionally bending the rules, even if it required a spiritual sacrifice. His gesture paid off, too, for my father would go on to become one of the country's top freestyle swimmers, and a member of the South African water polo team at the 1952 Summer Olympic Games in Helsinki. Later, he would run the foundation my maternal grandfather started and become a city councillor, determined to fight apartheid at the local level.

My mother, Estelle Mauerberger Yach, was a woman of her class and time, not coddled but accustomed to a standard of living that most people in South Africa could not begin to imagine. She loved her children, but wasn't quite sure what to do with us tiny, squawking mysteries whom she often left with a nanny and other servants. In her set, it was what one did back then. One of the images I carry of her from childhood is of a short, glamorous figure—wreathed in smoke, a lit Rothmans cigarette delicately held between nicotine-stained fingers, trailing ashes behind her. It was a part of her, Mother-and-Cigarette, Cigarette-and-Mother, all in one, our family's version of the Madonna-and-Child. She smoked at least thirty cigarettes a day for decades, unable to quit, not cold turkey and certainly not with the help of a nicotine patch, nicotine gum, or acupuncture.[2] It was the act that she loved, and the ritual. Lighting up and taking that first deep drag. Beside her always, an ashtray full of stubbed-out cigarette butts stained with lipstick, and I can still conjure her scent, a blend of perfume and smoke, fresh-blown overlaying stale. Many years later, when I was working on antitobacco campaigns as an epidemiologist in South Africa, she would show up at meetings I organized.

"Listen to my son," she told attendees. "He knows what he's talking about because he has lived with me—and I can't quit."

Mother began to smoke when she was a teenager, exiled with her three sisters to a boarding school in New Jersey, unhappy, and wanting only to come home. My grandfather—her father—had sent them to the United States during the Second World War so they would be safe from the burgeoning anti-Semitism that was sweeping South Africa. Nationalism was on the rise, with "Greyshirts" or *Gryshemde*—the name commonly given to the South African Gentile National Socialist Movement—marching openly in the streets and attacking those who were different. They were Nazis plain and simple, white thugs, their prejudice unleashed and inflamed by the Nazi movement in Germany. My grandfather himself had been set upon as he walked along the street near his home. Beaten with fists, truncheons, and jackboots, he ultimately lost an eye.

For four years, my mother and her sisters remained in New Jersey, only once venturing beyond its borders to a summer camp in Maine with rustic cabins, swimming, canoeing, kayaking, and lots of blackflies.

"I detested it," she told me many years later.

My three siblings—Dianna, Theodore, and Jonathan—and I would all grow up to be accomplished, engaged adults whom Mother is intensely proud of, but she was puzzled by us as children, perhaps because her own mother was chronically ill and died young. Her passion was collecting miniatures, and she spent much of her spare time creating tiny, perfect houses with tiny pieces of furniture and tiny doll residents who sat where she placed them, silent and obedient. They were her tableaux—idealized scenes of a yearned-for life. Of a life she could control.

Her father, my maternal grandfather Morris Mauerberger, was only fourteen when he arrived from Lithuania via London in 1904 to work with his older brother, Israel, in a fledgling drapery business. Despite little formal education, he was determined to make the best of his new country, cannily parlaying his first job peddling the company's dry goods door to door into a full-fledged textile company, then branching out to become a partner in a department store, and, finally, a property developer. Though he transformed himself from "Moshe" to "Morris," dapper and respected, he never forgot where he had come from and who he was: a member of a proud Jewish community that knew what it was like to be singled out and persecuted.

Despite the brutal attack that led to his sending his daughters away, my grandfather refused to leave, standing his ground and quietly responding to his tormenters by becoming even more successful, a powerful, rich businessman. He eventually started the Mauerberger Foundation Fund, which supported a number of wide-ranging causes, both Jewish and non-Jewish, as well as academic programs. One of its first endowments was for a chair in the school of ophthalmology at the University of Cape Town. It wasn't revenge for the loss of his eye that drove him so much as turning his experience into something positive to help countless others—because he could.

Although my parents were both first-generation offspring of Jews from Europe, the differences between them—in class and in religious observance—were so great that it was as if they came from two different worlds. Where my father's family shut their automotive repair shop near the edge of the city without fail for the Sabbath and kept a strictly kosher home, the Mauerbergers were non-observant Jews who went to synagogue only on the High Holy Days and had servants to attend to their every whim. Where he attended university for a year before quitting to go to work at his father's shop, she never finished high school, opting for some reason not to go back when she returned to Cape Town from the United States. Where he was fit and athletic, with broad shoulders and renowned in the Jewish community and beyond for his swimming prowess, she was quite overweight, until she had her first child, Dianna. From then on, she was fierce about remaining thin.

They were introduced to each other by my father's sister, my aunt Dorothy, who worked for Grandpa Morris as a secretary. Was it a match forged in love? I don't really know. Perhaps for my mother, it was a match at least partly made in rebellion against the strict social mores of the day, which dictated whom you dated and married. In her world, compared to more conventional Jewish boys she had dated, my father was exotic—a man of the working class, and an athlete, to boot. After they married, my father went to work for Grandpa Morris, eventually running the foundation and serving on the local council.

My parents kept their children at some distance when we were young. Maybe that was just their nature. Maybe my mother's upbringing dictated how we would be raised. Or perhaps they were unsure how to relate to small children, with whom they could not carry on conversations about the issues that sparked their passion and ire—racism, apartheid, the governing National Party pro-Afrikaner platform, and international sanctions that had been levied against the country. So they left us in the care of a nanny, a cook, a driver, and various other servants who kept watch over us and made sure we were doing our homework and not running roughshod over the neighborhood. It was a sheltered existence; radio broadcasts were controlled by the state and heavily censored, and television didn't come to the country until 1976. Hendrik Verwoerd, who served as prime minister from 1958 until he was assassinated in 1966, once even compared the medium to atomic bombs and poison gas, claiming that all three may be modern inventions but that didn't make them desirable.

"The government has to watch for any dangers to the people, both spiritual and physical," he said.

My strongest memories from early childhood were marked by swimming and weekend forays with my father to visit his family, where I sat and smiled because I did not speak Yiddish. Sometimes, we took long walks together on Sundays, which I loved, because I had him to myself and we could talk about anything I wanted, be it school, swimming, or life in general. Having to share my father with his demanding job, with my sister and younger brothers, with visitors to our house who wanted counsel and support, it was a selfish pleasure to have him all to myself.

"Respect and hard work is what it takes to succeed," he was wont to tell me. And "If you see something that is wrong, don't be silent."

We were privileged, to be sure, able to live in a park-like setting in a home that grew in size with us, with rooms and wings added as needed. My mother kept a room strictly for her miniature creations, off limits to all of us except Dianna, her only daughter. There were house servants and a chauffeur who doubled as our gardener—a way of life that came with a profound sense of obligation. For my father, that meant getting involved in politics and for my mother, volunteering for various Jewish charities. As children, we were instilled with a clear sense of right and wrong and the need to get involved and give back.

As I got older, my parents increasingly allowed me and Dianna into their lives; I listened to the conversation around their dinner table, with guests who were Jewish, Christian, Muslim, and Hindu, with skin that was black, white, and brown. The talk was heated and political, and for my family, at least, the pogroms of the late nineteenth and early twentieth centuries and the ovens of the Holocaust silently framed the discussion, as did the attack on my grandfather closer to home. How could we, as Jews, stand by and watch as others— Blacks, Coloureds, and Indians, as the government classified them—were segregated, oppressed, and sometimes killed?

How could anyone with a shred of human decency stand by as Blacks were forcibly removed from their homes and lost their South African citizenship in the process? The country, in its effort to ensure the all-time supremacy of Whites in the country, had become an isolated island full of hate, an outcast and anathema to the rest of the world.

Still, we stayed. Although many other South African Jewish families fled the country, for my family, there was no other option. We had to stay, to stand up against apartheid and fight from within to effect change. We loved South Africa, which had provided safe harbor to my grandparents from both sides. It was home, in all its physical beauty and political ugliness.

In grade eleven, I helped start our school's first-ever student council and debating union. Such organizations had been forbidden outright in the past, but even though the official end of apartheid was still twenty-odd years away, the African National Congress had begun to make waves that were increasingly being felt within South Africa's borders. The government needed to demonstrate to the world that they were open to *some* semblance of change. All of a sudden, we were debating the need for desegregation and ending apartheid, turning over moral and ethical issues as if discovering them for the first time. Some of us probably were. It was heady and scary all at once because we had to keep looking over our shoulders for authorities who could censor us, or worse if we were *too* rebellious or vociferous.

Adapt. Work within the system to change it. Growing up, it was one of the most important lessons I learned, along with the maxim to never give up, no matter how hard the going gets.

Upon entering medical school at the University of Cape Town in 1974, I became ever more involved in student dissent. I'd decided to become a doctor less from a desire to heal individual people and more from a need to be in a position to effect change on a grander scale. As vice president of the medical students' council—the education system in South Africa is set up so that one doesn't do an undergraduate degree before going on to study medicine—we fought for an end to apartheid, for an education system that was open to all, and a justice system that treated everyone equally, no matter their skin color. And then, Soweto happened and our world, already on shaky ground, was turned upside down.

On June 16, 1976, thousands of students in the sprawling Black township on the outskirts of Johannesburg walked to a rally at Orlando Stadium to protest a government decree that they be schooled in Afrikaans. Desmond Tutu, then the bishop of Lesotho, had called Afrikaans—a language that most Blacks did not speak—the language of the oppressor. The protest was supposed to be peaceful, with singing, speeches, and placards; when police blocked the route for one group of students, they found another way to get there. In the end, it didn't matter. The police opened fire on the crowd, on *kids*, who ran for their lives. By the next day, Soweto was on fire, with a pall of black smoke hanging over it. Rioters burned government buildings and police blundered in, firing into crowds at will. At least 176 people died, probably more. The government demanded that the names of those who came to emergency departments with gunshot wounds be handed over so they could be arrested and tried. Doctors refused, claiming they were treating "abscesses," not gunshot wounds.

The images haunt me still. Kids, many of them in black-and-white school uniforms, marching, their mouths open in song and peaceful protest. Placards with the handwritten messages "To hell with Afrikaans" and "Away with Afrikaans." Another read, "For freedom, we all lay down our lives." Worst of all, there was the photo of twelve-year-old Hector Pieterson, thin legs dangling and blood streaming from his mouth, lying lifeless in the arms of an older boy named Mbuyisa Makhubo. As Hector's older sister, Antoinette Sithole, runs alongside, crying, the anger and determination on Makhubo's face says it all. *This was a child. A child still young enough to wear shorts. And you, the police, cut him down.*

Despite the government's best efforts, the photo was published and the gaping, festering sore—the *abscess*—at the heart of our country was there for all the world to see. In that moment, I realized I had to do something more, and began to think about what my role in the revolution should be. For there *would* be a revolution, and rather than become a doctor, with a hazy, feel-good idea of healing the world, I thought maybe it would be better to study law, as my older sister was doing, and to take on human rights cases. I broached the subject with my father. He said: "That's all well and fine. I'd be very happy for you to pursue a career in law—after you finish medical school."

Unspoken was the lesson he'd taught me all those years ago: *Be brave. Be tough. Take risks, don't give up and, most of all, don't be afraid to fail.*

Back at university, protest became a major part of our lives. We marched. We monitored human rights violations and we published pamphlets, including a medical newsletter I edited with the woman who would become my wife, Yasmin von Schirnding. We had to be careful that our stories about the system didn't fall completely afoul of the laws at the time. For the authorities, everything was suspect, whether articles that promoted health for all or detailed inequities in how the government provided health services. A whispered criticism of the government could get you arrested, while being found in possession of publications such as Mao Tse-tung's *Little Red Book*, with its aphorisms like "Political power grows out of the barrel of a gun," could get you tossed in jail.

While the university itself was antiapartheid and made sure its classes were desegregated, it was driven home to us on a daily basis how the system held non-Whites back. In hospitals, for example, where government regulations prevailed, white students like me got to treat patients on both the Coloured and White wards, but Coloured students could only treat Coloured patients. It was limiting—and an insult that made me more determined than ever to somehow bring about change.

In 1978, the primary health care movement was launched during a World Health Organization (WHO) conference in Alma-Ata (now Almaty), Kazakhstan, which ended with the proclaimed lofty goal of "Health for All by the Year 2000."[3] Excited and inspired, we monitored the talks and wrote about them extensively. Addressing the health needs of all had a haunting resonance in South Africa, with its downtrodden populations, and there were times when we felt we had to speak out, no matter the risk. We established the Koeberg Alert, about a nuclear power station that was being built on the doorstep of a mixed-race community 18.5 miles north of Cape Town that had no electricity. How would the South African government deal with the radioactive waste? Was this the first building block in an attempt by the country to become a nuclear power? And why locate it there? It was at around the same time that the Three Mile Island nuclear power plant in Dauphin County, Pennsylvania, had had a partial meltdown. It was this, above all, that incensed us. If there was a leak—or worse, a meltdown—the community's residents would suffer the full brunt of an evacuation and any medical fallout, yet they did not benefit from the cheaper power source down the road.

Where, we wondered, was the justice in *that*?

■

As a medical intern, I spent a year working in pediatric surgery and general medical clinics. I hadn't been there long when I began to question out loud whether or not Black patients were being fully informed before agreeing to take part in clinical research trials. The superintendent of hospitals, Dr. Hannah-Reeve Sanders—a brave woman who nonetheless had to abide by the rules—worried that we were politicizing the role of interns and that this would cause problems for us in the future. I'm not sure if it did or not, but it didn't matter to me anyway. For the first time in my career as a young doctor, I saw how I could make a difference in a country going through political upheaval. Through my work with patients, I could help a whole population.

When I graduated in 1979, I had to make a choice: compulsory service in the South African Army (which had been deferred while I was at medical school), jail as a conscientious objector, or fleeing the country. Some of my classmates left. One close friend went to jail.

Like my parents and my grandparents, even though I hated the apartheid system, I loved South Africa. I loved the open countryside, the sand dunes that bloomed in the spring, and Table Mountain looming over Cape Town, with scrub grass, goats, and a flat top often covered in what looked like lacework spun from clouds. Although my father discouraged open-sea swimming because it was so risky—for him, pools and races were the way to go—I loved powering through the Atlantic Ocean, through waves and changing tides, from

Clifton to Barker Rock, from Simon's Town, where the Indian Ocean meets the Atlantic, to Muizenberg. Later, I made the 6.5-mile swim from Three Anchor Bay to Robben Island, where the prison was once home to people like Nelson Mandela and Jacob Zuma—an official event that would become known as the "Long Swim to Freedom."

I had a connection here, and goals. Like my parents, I decided to stay and serve in the army.

At the same time, Dr. Marian Jacobs, a senior lecturer, fantastic clinician, and later dean of the university's medical school, realized before I did that, with my interests and tendency to agitate, I should specialize in epidemiology and public health. She sent me to the South African Medical Research Council (SAMRC) to meet Dr. Hannes Botha, who was researching and documenting health inequalities in the country.

Actually, she said, "Do your patients a favor, Derek, and go into epidemiology. *Please.*"

That June, I began a double-header of a job, studying epidemiology at the SAMRC while undergoing military training and completing an officer's course. Afterwards, I was shipped off, first to a rural hospital and then to the Namibian border in the north. This was because, in October 1975, the country had become embroiled in a Cold War proxy war in Angola, where, after gaining independence from Portugal, various factions were fighting for control. South Africa supported the National Union for the Total Independence of Angola (UNITA), but really, it was West versus East, the United States and countries such as ours against the Soviet Union and its allies, including Cuba.

When I finally got to the dry, dusty Namibian border, I announced that I was "noncombatant."

Staff at the makeshift hospital laughed. "That's a pretty stupid position, Doctor," I was told. "You can say that all you want, but you know what? They're going to shoot you anyway!"

Throughout this period, I kept up my swimming every day, climbing into a big tank filled with dirty water and doing laps. The orderlies would help me by stretching surgical tubing across the tank to create a lane I could follow even when I was doing backstroke, back and forth for at least thirty minutes, longer when I was not needed at the makeshift hospital.

At night, I rode in helicopters across the border, landing in forsaken areas to pick up wounded fighters, mostly Cubans, and trying to make sure they stayed alive until they got back to the hospital. With the rotors, it was loud, making it difficult for me to listen for a beating heart or breaths. Most of them didn't make it. I can still conjure the smell of their blood, salty and metallic—a memory that can assault me when I least expect it. I was watching TV news footage in 2013 of the Boston Marathon bombings and their aftermath when, all of a sudden, I was back in a helicopter, spattered in blood and smelling it everywhere—and I began to cry.

Then, there was the torture. I won't—I can't—go into it without feeling sick to my stomach, but I did write a letter to my commanding officer that described the callous acts I'd witnessed. Within a few days of having sent that letter, I was whisked away on a plane with blacked-out windows and transferred to a military hospital in Cape Town. I hadn't realized that all letters written from the border were opened and screened for content, even those from officers. Mine, with its incendiary accusations, was quickly hushed up.

At first, the hospital was a good place to work. In between shifts on the wards, I was able to start an informal epidemiology study down in the naval dockyard, looking at asbestos-related diseases such as mesothelioma, a cancer for which there is no cure. The rate of occurrence was higher among those who worked in submarines and in the boilermakers inside ships. But when I asked to do a more formal study, the military said, "No thanks—and please stop what you're doing *now*."

I was disappointed, but Botha, my mentor at the SAMRC, continued to stress the importance of looking at health issues from a different perspective—one based on data but still able to zero in on singular human experience. He emphasized critical thinking and problem-based understanding; early on, we focused on documenting the discrepancy in life expectancies in South Africa and noticed that the amount and quality of data for the Black population was deficient, at best.

In the mid-1980s, I left South Africa to complete a master's in public health at Johns Hopkins University in Baltimore, spending fifteen months in that city. It was the most exhilarating time, but I missed my girlfriend, Yasmin, whom I would marry in 1987 in the garden of my parents' home—and I never lost sight of the fact that I was training to take on the battle back in my own country. That I wanted, that I *needed*, to fight from within.

■

In 1985, I returned to a country in chaos. Black townships burned amidst violent protests against the lack of services and facilities. Rocks were thrown from freeways, tires burned, and mines exploded. In a suburb of Port Elizabeth, police opened fire on a crowd gathered to commemorate the twenty-fifth anniversary of the Sharpeville Massacre. In Cape Town, more than two hundred people were arrested as they marched to call for Nelson Mandela's release from Pollsmoor Prison.

Amidst all of this, I went to the SAMRC boss, Dr. Andries Brink, a bespectacled cardiologist who had served as dean of the medical faculty at Stellenbosch University and was vilified by some as a government yes-man who didn't like to make waves. Young and passionate, I wanted to make a big one.

"As an epidemiologist, I think it's our responsibility to document the effect of political violence on health," I said, a bit nervous. "It's important as a research council to demonstrate this without having to get political about it."

I half-expected him to cut me off mid-sentence. To say something like "The government won't hear of it." Or "Yach, you should know by now what we can and can't do. So, no way."

To my surprise, he said, "Yes."

I was given a grant of about 30,000 rand—a fortune back then—which allowed us to look at the daily lives of people in 1,540 households in neighborhoods with varying degrees of violence; at the lives of nurses struggling to deliver health care in high-violence areas; and at the disruption the violence caused to the delivery of basic services such as water, street lights, sanitation, and transportation. We also found that the number of gunshot wounds in high-impact areas was three times higher than in low-impact ones.

Concerned that authorities would be able to access SAMRC files, get the names of those they had shot, and then arrest them, and having learned from my previous military experience that little is private, I asked the South African Red Cross Society to supervise the study. If authorities did seize the files from this arm of a respected international, nonprofit, and charitable organization, there would be a huge international outcry.

Two years later, the study was published in the *American Journal of Public Health*.[4] It was a proud moment, in no small measure because, outside of South Africa, people—my peers included—had always tended to see white South Africans as oppressors, simply because of the color of our skin. If I was white, because I was white, I had to be bad, because I continued to live and work in a country shunned by the rest of the world for its racist policies. Our papers were turned down by most other leading journals outside the country and some

conferences barred us from attending. The result was that
South Africa was behind when it came to medical advance-
ment; when we did get to travel to conferences, we absorbed
masses of information at every opportunity, cramming in as
many sessions as we could, reeling from one to the next from
early morning until late at night.

Brink and I never spoke about why he agreed to the survey
in the first place. But in hindsight, I like to think he was a
pragmatist, a closemouthed man who in the end did not close
his mind to what was happening around him. Perhaps he
saw a future when Blacks would live among Whites, and
maybe—probably—even run the country. And maybe he felt
the transition would be smoother if we were able to gather as
much information as possible beforehand, to listen to people's
stories and be in a position to respond. He couldn't have
foreseen that the survey might help to bring down barriers
between the South African medical establishment and the rest
of the world, which had shunned us as white professionals
in a country run by a racist regime. But in the end, that is
what it did.

In 1989, as the African National Congress consolidated its
power and profile, Brink pulled me aside. In a sop to the international community, the apartheid government was going to
allow Blacks to move into cities. But before that happened,

we were being asked to conduct a study that would assure Whites they would not die of infection.

"You're kidding, right?" I asked, even though I knew he wasn't.

Later, meeting with Hannes Botha and another SAMRC colleague, Lucy Wagstaff, we knew there was no way we were going to do it. How could we do a study that catered to racist White fears about the Black majority? Instead, we decided that what was really needed was an official center for epidemiological research that addressed *all* major health problems in the country—from HIV/AIDS and malaria to violence—in a more systematic, clinical way. In turn, we hoped that would lead to the creation of a national health program that optimized how we looked at the health benefits and pitfalls of urbanization in the first place.

We were going to do the unthinkable: stand up to authority. In the proposal, we were blunt about what we wanted and why. To my surprise (again!), Brink didn't question us at all. Instead, he quietly redirected the money into what would become the Center for Epidemiological Research in South Africa (CERSA) and he asked me to be its director.

Finally, we were cleared to do what I'd dreamed of all along: work toward health for all in South Africa. We looked at the impact of urbanization, starting with Soweto, and we worked on improving immunization rates, strengthened tuberculosis control, and instituted more effective treatment of traumatic brain injuries from violence and motor vehicle accidents. We looked at noncommunicable diseases, too, including the rise of type 2 diabetes, cardiovascular conditions, and cancer.

Once again, it proved the lesson I had learned from my father long before. That first swim in my grandfather's pool was a watery rite of passage, a calculated lesson in confidence, courage, and can-do. I have applied that lesson over and over again in all aspects of my life. No matter how rough the water gets. It is as if my father is there, whispering in my ear: *Be brave. Be tough. Take risks, don't give up and, most of all, don't be afraid to fail.*

2

FINDING
MY WAY

I can't remember a time when I didn't hate the smell of cigarettes, how the secondhand smoke made my throat burn and my clothes stink. I hated it when my mother and her sisters would all light up. Later, I hated what I knew it was doing to their hearts and their lungs, turning them from a healthy pink to black. The link between smoking and lung cancer had been established as early as 1949. By the time I was in medical school, and despite the tobacco companies' denials—lies—that there was anything wrong, we knew the risk in excruciating wheezing-coughing-choking detail. We saw the cancer-ridden lungs preserved in jars for medical research, disfigured by irregularly shaped black tumors, and we knew there was precious little we could do to stem the progression of tobacco-related disease once it had begun. Whenever I walked past someone who was smoking, I would cough exaggeratedly and wave my hands in disgust, as if to sweep the smoker from my surroundings. Except for my mother. If I wanted to see her, I had to suffer her smoking, holding my breath and my tongue.

My antitobacco campaigning began in earnest in my last year of university, where smoking was permitted everywhere but in classrooms. Frustrated, a group of us on the medical students' council developed an antitobacco campaign that highlighted the science and the scary statistics.

Before launching it, we decided to get the full picture by paying a visit to the Rembrandt Tobacco Corporation, an Afrikaans-owned multinational company that, despite worldwide condemnation of apartheid, the South African government was able to tout as an international success story. We didn't think the visit through terribly clearly. We were young and we wanted to challenge them. We wanted to give them a chance to explain why they were doing what they did and to respond to our campaign, which highlighted the numbers of deaths from tobacco-related causes such as cancer and heart disease.

Known outside the country as Rothmans International, Rembrandt had been founded in 1948 by Anton Rupert, an erstwhile medical student turned chemistry major who owned a dry-cleaning business before going into something much more lucrative.

Rembrandt had a long history of backing the National Party, which was dominated by Afrikaans-speaking South Africans. The two were, in fact, founded in the same year, 1948, and grew up together, feeding off each other. The company paid for annual outings for Cabinet ministers; in its turn, the government refused to restrict smoking in public places and to censor advertising in any way, and it kept excise taxes low. Rupert himself was one of the most powerful businessmen in the country, with a seat on the boards of most major trusts and with powerful cronies in government, media, and law. It would not be long before I would discover just how powerful Rupert was, how long the reach of his power. But on that day, we were young, idealistic students off to confront a power broker, come what may.

I traveled by car with Chris Hugo Hamman, my closest childhood friend and soon-to-be Rhodes Scholar, to Stellenbosch, about thirty-one miles east of Cape Town, where Rembrandt—originally called *Voorbrand*, the Afrikaans word for "fire-break"—had its headquarters. Despite our belief that we were doing the right thing by giving the other side the chance to explain itself, we were so nervous as we stepped into the building! It looked rich and clean. Wood floors gleamed, art hung on white walls, and, rarest of all, workers of all races— Black, Coloured, and White—greeted us. It was a perfect show of solidarity, a sign that Rembrandt did not discriminate. Anton Rupert, the big man himself, escorted us into a boardroom with a large wooden table, its surface polished to a high gloss. A bowl of apples had been placed on it, not quite within our reach. We sat down. Rupert immediately gestured with his arm at the closed door.

"We're better employers of Blacks than anybody else in the country," he said without preamble. "We invest in national heritage and our environmental policies are cutting edge."

Cautiously, I replied: "All that is great, but it doesn't take away from the fact that your product is killing people."

Rupert's answer was at once infuriating and, sadly, not unexpected. "Tobacco is not having an impact on health in South Africa because there are so many other health problems," he said.

In response, all we could do was point to the horrific statistics on smoking and health in other parts of the world. Truth be told, at the time, there *was* very little data on the effect of tobacco within South Africa's borders, and the tobacco companies themselves were overseeing the few studies being done and keeping the results to themselves. However, we believed the studies would emphasize freedom of choice over health problems. And the country *did* have lots of health problems other than tobacco-related conditions, from malaria to chronic malnutrition among the Black population, and asbestos-related diseases such as mesothelioma, an aggressive cancer that was—and still is—a death sentence.

Nonetheless, we thought tobacco companies shouldn't get away with producing a product that kills just because Blacks worked for them, or because they planted trees, supported symphony orchestras, or provided Christmas baskets to the poor. It was akin to saying you should be allowed to sell alcohol because you produced good oranges, which didn't make sense at all.

We drove back to Cape Town convinced we were right. At least, that is what we told each other. Soon after, we launched the UCT Anti-Tobacco Campaign, with professionally produced posters and a lot of statistics. As far as campaigns go, it wasn't terribly effective, but our meeting with Rupert taught us an important lesson that would guide us for the rest of our lives: there was a need to gather statistics on the toll of smoking in South Africa that were independent of politicians and companies with their own interests at play. And it marked the official start of my own campaign against Big Tobacco and the damage its products wreak on individuals, families, and society as a whole.

I had found my way to make a difference.

■

When I graduated, I found work at the SAMRC, heeding the wise advice offered to me years earlier by Marian Jacobs, that my strengths lay in epidemiological research rather than by the bedsides of ailing patients. My first project, which I did while preparing for military service, was a study of the economic aspects of smoking in the country. It was controversial, to say the least. I showed that, rather than stressing the need to reduce tobacco and cigarette production as the key to reducing consumption, the South African Medical Association, along with the national apartheid government, emphasized education programs, which had little effect, if any. Which may have been the point. After all, the tobacco industry was an integral part of the country's economy and any reduction would mean a loss of revenue on every level— for government, business and the people who worked in both worlds.

I worked hard, collating the best data I could (including some sent to me by a Rembrandt manager!). But in the end, the council declined to allow me to publish my paper under the SAMRC banner, probably because it contained statistics that starkly showed the effects of tobacco consumption on the health—and deaths—of South Africans. Perhaps the pressures were just too great.

Despite Rembrandt's efforts to quell any news that was not positive, I was unwilling to give up. In 1982, I submitted the paper to the *South African Medical Journal* on my own, using my home address in the Claremont neighborhood of Cape Town. The journal published it the following year. Titled the "Economic Aspects of Smoking in South Africa," the paper got a huge amount of publicity and went on to win an award as one of the medical research papers of the year.[5]

Four years later, in 1987, the World Health Organization (WHO) was planning to launch a "World No Tobacco Day" on April 7, 1988. At that time, South Africa was still under sanctions and barred from joining entities such as WHO, but I was fascinated by the organization and visited whenever I could get the government to grant me a permit to leave the country. I developed contacts and friends and dreamed of one day working there.

When I learned of this initiative, I was so inspired that I convinced the editor of the *South African Medical Journal* to publish a special edition in 1988 devoted entirely to tobacco control and linked to the international event.[6] It was the first time the journal had ever devoted an entire issue to a preventive aspect of public health, and it was a critical turning point. Rather than simply warn that deaths would increase, we were able to project exactly what would happen in the future and show that other countries around the world had passed laws to stem the damage. Both were considered a major breakthrough in tobacco control.

The mass media picked up the issue and ran with it. Using the dense epidemiological data that until then had languished in scientific journals, media painted a more graphic picture that the public could understand and identify with: what a death from lung cancer looked like, what secondhand smoke could do to loved ones, and how marketing was geared to their own children with the goal of hooking them for life, for however long that life lasted. And very significantly, Brink, who was still the president of the SAMRC, wrote a powerful editorial of support despite the rejection of my paper a few years before.[7]

I considered the journal issue a first sortie, a testing of the waters. The question was whether it would affect public perception and lead to government action beyond education programs. Would it lead to actual tobacco controls?

The answer? Yes, and no. At first, F.W. de Klerk, the country's president at the time, announced he was working on as-yet-unspecified changes to legislation, which made us hopeful, but the changes remained unspecified until they disappeared altogether. A 1989 editorial in the *South African Medical Journal* took Rembrandt's Rupert to task for using fuzzy, emotive language to obscure unpleasant facts, including that nearly half the patients at Groote Schuur, a primary care hospital in Cape Town, suffered from tobacco-related diseases, from lung cancer to heart failure.[8] In March 1989, my former medical school, which used the hospital as a training ground, banned smoking and the sale of cigarettes in all public areas, including the campus's restaurants and bars.

I savored that small victory.

But popular opinion remained split, the old guard versus the new, smokers balking at change versus doctors, scientists, and those who wanted to live a healthier lifestyle. Sometimes, the fighting got vicious—the "civilized" adult version of a bare-knuckles brawl in a school yard. In 1989, when Cape Town's city council announced a vote on a proposal put forth by the city's chief medical officer to limit cigarette advertising and smoking in public places, Anton Rupert responded by threatening to withdraw Rembrandt's sponsorship of the

Cape Town Philharmonic Orchestra. It was a bully tactic and it worked.

Still, there were signs that his influence was on the wane, the most glaring being that the majority of council members voted in favor of the proposal. In the end, Kobus Meiring, administrator of Cape Province, caved to pressure and refused to pass legislation needed for the council to enforce its plans.

On the national level, the tide began to turn when Carole Charlewood, an opposition member of Parliament and former TV personality, charged the government with "protecting the vested interests of the powerful tobacco industry, and not the people of the country."[9] She based the charge on the 1988 report I co-wrote for the SAMRC entitled "Smoking in South Africa: The Need for Action," in which we warned that the costs of the tobacco industry outweighed its benefits.

Rina Venter, health minister in de Klerk's last Cabinet (and the first woman in South Africa to serve in Cabinet, period), responded right away, promising to look into tobacco control legislation. Her Cabinet colleagues weren't happy but there it was: an undertaking by a Cabinet minister in a government with close ties to the tobacco industry. True to her word, a draft bill was introduced in March 1992. Two months later, on May 31—the fifth annual World No Tobacco Day—Nelson Mandela, who had been released from prison in 1990 after serving twenty-seven years behind bars, declared his full support for the draft bill and went even further, calling for all South Africans to support antitobacco campaigns.

We had come a long way—but we weren't quite there yet. Change would come. It *was* coming. Apartheid was coming to an end and, with it, the influence of people like Rupert.

■

By the end of 1990, with Mandela set free, South Africa was fast becoming a darling of the development world. With the help of grants from the US-based Henry J. Kaiser Family Foundation, those who were exiled by the apartheid regime began to return, first in a trickle, then a flood. They came to get to know their country again before they took their place in government, to familiarize themselves with the structures in place. At the SAMRC, we were fortunate to work with people such as Dr. Nkosazana Dlamini-Zuma, who in 1994 would become the first health minister in Mandela's Government of National Unity.

Taking advantage of this new openness, in 1992, I approached Zimbabwe's minister of health, Timothy Stamps, to help me organize the first-ever Africa conference on tobacco control. I wanted to tweak and push, and Stamps, who'd been born in Wales and trained as a doctor in the United Kingdom before moving to colonial Rhodesia in 1962 to join the public health service, was the perfect partner to help do it. He was smart, fearless, and farsighted. Fired by the public health service in 1974, allegedly for skewing health care services to Blacks over Whites, he didn't return to the United Kingdom.

Instead, he continued to work as a doctor, to build clinics, and to agitate on behalf of communities that were underserviced. As health minister in the new Zimbabwean government, he trumpeted as his slogan "Health for All by the Year 2000" and oversaw a major expansion of public health services.

For a year, we met in secret at a rugby stadium in Pretoria, South Africa—to anyone watching, just two white men in casual clothes and sunglasses, arms crossed over our chests as we pretended to watch the matches. We couldn't let people in power learn of the conference too far in advance. Although a transitional government was in place in South Africa, the situation was still politically delicate, and Zimbabwe happened to be one of the largest tobacco-growing centers in the world. The tobacco companies would be most unhappy, as would the farmers, when they learned what we were doing.

"We need to show them we aren't against them," Stamps said, his arms folded as he pretended to idly watch the match.

We sat there, through game after game, week after week, passing back and forth papers and suggestions for topics and guests. Quietly, we had obtained funding from the International Research Development Centre in Canada, the Swedish International Development Cooperation Agency, the US government, the World Bank, and the Rockefeller Foundation. Former US president Jimmy Carter had recorded a video address that urged world leaders to support the Africa conference. When we finally scheduled it for November 14–17, 1993, in Harare, Zimbabwe, it was exciting. People from thirty countries would be represented, and our guests would include the world's top experts, such as Dr. Ruth Roemer of UCLA, a pioneer in public health law.

Once news of the conference was finally made public, the tobacco companies, unbeknownst to us, unleashed a plot to sabotage it. In early October, United Tobacco Company Ltd. (a subsidiary of British American Tobacco [BAT]) organized a conference for select journalists to be held just before ours at an exclusive, luxurious resort in South Africa. The invitation stated that independent international experts would give seminars to allegedly correct misconceptions about the alleged health effects of tobacco, the effects of advertising on tobacco usage and the activities of the World Health Organization. Among those experts was Dr. Sharon Boyse, the head of BAT's smoking issues department, who argued there was no medical evidence of smoking's ill health effects, and Dr. Jean Boddewyn of Baruch College in New York City, whose lecture about the effects of advertising on smoking behavior was actually paid for by the International Advertising Association.

That wasn't all. In the weeks leading up to the conference, a pre-emptive publicity campaign by tobacco companies in Zimbabwe framed our conference as a threat to the country and a cause of extreme alarm to the world's tobacco manufacturers. A newspaper article in *The Farmer* noted: "One thing is certain: the conference will attract a wide cross section of the anti-smoking industry's groupies who are known to be particularly virulent, if not necessarily well-informed."[10]

Anti-smoking "industry"? Groupies? It was an interesting way to describe our efforts to save people's lives—and
to think of describing people such as Roemer as a groupie
beggared belief. Intense and charismatic, she had fought
to expand women's reproductive rights in California, cam-
paigned for fluoride to be added to water supplies across the
United States and was now on the warpath against tobacco.
She was dynamic, devoted to her work, and a mesmerizing
speaker. A groupie she was not.

Indeed, at the conference, it was Roemer whose speech
openly called for an international treaty approach to tobacco.
In a few moments, she managed to encapsulate what I had
been working toward for my whole career as an epidemiologist
with an interest in prevention and a master's in public health.

From my vantage point at the SAMRC and as co-organizer
of the conference, it seemed history was happening on our
watch, with the flag planted in Harare.

■

As a medical student and then as an epidemiologist, I'd always
been fascinated by WHO. But as a white South African, it was
difficult for me to visit the organization and make contacts
who could help us in our efforts to effect change in South
Africa. But Mandela's release from prison in 1990 helped to
release us, too. That year, I arranged the first trip by South
African medical researchers to WHO's regional headquarters

for Africa, located in Brazzaville, in the Republic of the Congo. From that moment on, I traveled as much as I could, from Cape Town to Geneva and beyond, meeting experts, cultivating relationships, showing them what we had done to combat various communicable and noncommunicable diseases, and trying to apply everything I was learning back at home.

Then, in 1995, I got the call from WHO to come to Geneva and become the first South African since apartheid ended to work there. It wasn't an easy choice, leaving the country I loved. I had chosen to remain and fight apartheid policies from the classroom and the medical front lines for the rights of every person—Black, Coloured, White, young, old, and disabled—to proper, full health care services. When I thought of it, I didn't really want to leave. I was perfectly glad to stay put, now that South Africa was in the world's good books again. As my parents and grandparents had taught me, I had a responsibility to stay and, with my colleagues, effect change on a grand scale where it was sorely needed. Yasmin was there, as was her family—and mine. And the country *was* changing. It felt like South Africa was on the brink of a great experiment that would either succeed or fail in spectacular fashion.

But the job offer at WHO presented such a rare opportunity for me to expand on preventive health work I was already doing in South Africa.

In the end, after many late-night discussions with Yasmin, we decided to go. After ten years together, we finally got married in my grandfather's garden, amid my father's threats to recite the Mourner's Kaddish—the Jewish prayer for the dead—because she wasn't Jewish. His opposition was one of the reasons it took us a decade to decide to marry. But in the end, he didn't recite the prayer at the ceremony and he soon came to love her, showing me yet again the importance of remaining open to ideas and people you may initially be uncomfortable with.

A few years later, I would learn the tobacco companies were creepily tracking my every move. Following my WHO appointment, a fax dated June 6, 1995, from Shabanji Opukah, a BAT employee, to all the company's public affairs managers in Africa stated:

> *Although Dr. Yach's office says this appointment has nothing to do with smoking or tobacco, my early basic research seems to indicate the contrary. I would therefore advise that we all be on the alert for a possible increase in the activities and influence of the WHO in Africa.*
>
> *Dr. Yach's ascendancy must have a lot to do with his anti-tobacco campaigns ... Added to the recent appointment of South Africa as the new external auditors to WHO, this only helps to enhance Africa's profile in the organization, which Dr. Yach will exploit to suit his well known anti-tobacco agenda.*[11]

In another fax, it is clear that information about me had been exchanged between Opukah at BAT and Hilary Thomson, corporate affairs manager for United Tobacco Company Ltd., an international tobacco-leaf business based in North Carolina. Opukah wrote:

> *His interests cover such aspects as the impact of smoking, the economic impact of the industry, smoking in black and coloured communities, advertising and restrictions in restaurants ... We need to keep track of all the developments by him if only to be able to know in advance what his next moves on restrictions are likely to be and then determine what we could do about such in advance.*
>
> *You may also be interested to know that as a professional and academic hardly in his mid career, the doctor is already very highly regarded and is seen as a high flier. I also understand that he has a relative or two who are smokers.[12]*

There was just one more thing I needed to do before leaving. In June 1995, a month before Yasmin and I moved from Cape Town to the little apartment in Nyon, Switzerland, that would be our home for the next seven years as we commuted into Geneva, I found myself back on the road to Rembrandt's headquarters in Stellenbosch. It was hot and dry, typical weather for that time of year. But this time, there would be no Anton Rupert to greet me. Instead, closing the circle I had begun as a medical student twenty years earlier, I was meeting Johann Rupert, who had taken over from his father as CEO. I wanted to know if the son was different: if he was open to change; if he recognized that the world was changing around him.

The answer came before we even spoke a word. Six feet tall, with a paunch and thick brown hair that framed a pale face, he stood waiting at the front of the classic Cape Dutch–style, white-stucco building that housed his office, a lit cigarette held at his side. For the whole of our forty-minute meeting, he never stopped stubbing out one, then lighting another: a silent message that no matter what I thought or what laws were passed, he was unrepentant.

He spent much of our time together complaining that stronger tobacco control regulations undermined the people's right to choose. I tried to counter him but soon realized there was no point. As I got ready to leave, I told him that I would soon be leaving the country for Geneva and WHO.

"Good," he said, puffing away. "You'll be out of my hair."

I smiled. "You're not getting rid of me at all," I said. "I'm going to globalize what I've been doing here for the last twenty years. I'm going to go global with my expertise."

He looked surprised. I might have, too. Even though it may have sounded like a bit of puffery and angling for position, I suddenly realized delivering that message was the reason I had come back to Rembrandt.

I was throwing down the gauntlet.

3

LEAVING HOME

I landed in Geneva at the end of summer 1995 to start my job, renting an apartment in nearby Nyon. Yasmin, who had a job lined up at WHO in environmental health, joined me six months later. We marvelled at the differences between this pristine city and Cape Town, at how people took their safety for granted and everything was on time, at the sheer tidiness of it and the plethora of food choices in the markets. Unlike in South Africa, most people spoke English, although German, French, and Italian were the official languages. Soon, I had a network of local swimming pools that I frequented and work colleagues who became friends.

Work was my focus, although it would be three years before I could make my mark in international tobacco control, three years before I would be named director of WHO's Tobacco Free Institute and become involved in the creation of the international tobacco control treaty. My first project at WHO was to renew and update for the twenty-first century WHO's Health for All policy, which had had its start at the Alma-Ata conference we had so closely monitored seventeen years earlier. To compile the Health for All report,[13] we were a group of four: Dr. Claire Chollat-Traquet, who I'd met when I was still in South Africa; Fernando Antezana; Dr. Douglas Bettcher, who I recruited; and me. We were tasked with reviewing the major health threats the world faced, identifying what diseases were being ignored or neglected, and how medical and technological advances provided new opportunities for treatment. The conclusion would be an extensive list of recommendations to be followed in order to create a new holistic policy.

Although it was a massive project that spoke to my passion for preventive health and instigating change, it would prove difficult to gain traction in an organization where the leadership and a lumbering bureaucracy did not consider our work a priority. It was frustrating because from the start, it was clear to us that the world was going through a major shift on the disease landscape. For much of the twentieth century, the major threat to world health was from communicable diseases such as hepatitis, malaria, and tuberculosis. But as the century waned, the threat from noncommunicable, chronic diseases grew—diseases where the risk factors included alcohol consumption, obesity, and tobacco use. Deadly conditions, such as emphysema and heart disease, type 2 diabetes, lung cancer and liver failure, didn't distinguish between First World and Third World, except in onset of disease, treatment options, and availability. In developing countries, disease tended to occur at a younger age, leading to longer periods of ill health, lost work hours, and premature death. In 2011, the World Bank would publish a report about noncommunicable diseases that cited one example after another, including the situation in Egypt, where the country's aggregate labor supply was 19 per cent under its potential because of workers who suffer from chronic conditions.[14] But in the mid- to late 1990s, we were already seeing the numbers, which should have raised the alarm in the highest echelons of WHO. Our report should have been a call to action. After years of being largely ignored, noncommunicable diseases should have been given the highest profile of all. Coming from South Africa, where I had worked with the best of the medical community to promote prevention, successfully taking on my superiors and the government, I was ready to make the reduction of these diseases my mission. But I was stymied by WHO's labyrinthine bureaucracy under the man at the top: Dr. Hiroshi Nakajima.

When he first came to WHO in 1973, Nakajima, a Japanese national who had studied in Paris and Tokyo, accomplished a lot. As the director of the organization's Drug Policies and Management unit, for example, he played a key role in developing the concept of essential medicines—drugs that health care professionals deem a priority for all countries. The list is regularly updated, and the drugs, which include lidocaine, morphine, and propofol, must be easily available and stored in enough quantities so that the supply never runs out.

Nakajima served as director-general from 1988 to 1998. His tenure was marked by a dispute with Dr. Jonathan Mann, a pioneer in the fight against AIDS-related diseases and the extraordinarily effective founding director of the organization's Global Programme on AIDS, who ended up resigning his position. Then it was our turn, and although we demonstrated repeatedly that noncommunicable diseases, from obesity to lung cancer, were proliferating throughout the world, we found ourselves sidelined—forgotten siblings toiling away in a division that was largely invisible to the rest of the organization. Most of the noncommunicable disease department heads and staff were straight out of the Cold War, politburo types from the Soviet Union who managed with little funding because they were accustomed to it and didn't do much work at all. And the head of the tobacco control department was a lovely man named Dr. Raúl Menchaca, a Cuban who happened to love smoking cigars.

Indeed, under Nakajima, WHO practically absolved itself of any responsibility to do anything with tobacco control, period, stating that it was something that required coordination by United Nations agencies in concert with each other. The man who was given responsibility to coordinate a response was an official with the United Nations Conference on Trade and

Development, a sister agency to WHO. He was a great guy, a lovely, gentle man and an observant Catholic who did not do much to make tobacco control policy a focal point for the United Nations as a whole. It was an egregious example of someone having a big title with no responsibility—and no one to call him on that fact!

Despite all this, there was a rustling, stealthy at first, from academics and WHO staff members, to change that attitude. Soon, it would get much louder.

■

The early to mid-1990s were a rockier time for tobacco companies than ever before. Although the deleterious effects of smoking had been known for decades, this period saw an important shift in the kinds of lawsuits that were filed around the world. Before, we saw a slew of cases in which individuals claimed damages because they had contracted cancer. Now, we were seeing class action suits begin to work their way through the courts, and cases where the attorneys general of various states based their arguments on the allegation that tobacco companies were guilty of engaging in racketeering and conspiracy. In addition, there was the fallout from the excruciating death of Wayne McLaren, a rodeo rider and smoker whose craggily handsome face became synonymous with cigarettes in the famous Marlboro Man ads. His last act before dying from lung cancer was to appear in an anti-smoking TV commercial that interspersed images of him as the cool cowboy with those of him lying wasted and unrecognizable in his hospital bed.

Around the world, tobacco advertising and sponsorships were taking hits, including in Australia, where the *Tobacco Advertising Prohibition Act* forbade almost all forms of tobacco advertising and new sponsorships.

In 1992, Allyn Taylor, a prickly, brilliant doctoral candidate of laws at Columbia University in New York City, published a groundbreaking paper in the *American Journal of Law & Medicine*.[15] In it, she argued that WHO had the constitutional authority to use unspecified legal mechanisms to reach the lofty goal of "Health for Everyone by the Year 2000." The paper caught the eye of Ruth Roemer, the powerhouse professor at UCLA's School of Public Health. In 1993, she met with Taylor, and together, they drew up a proposal for a formal international convention, or treaty, on tobacco use in order to advance the cause of public health.

That same year, Roemer, a former smoker who turned to pipes before giving up the habit altogether in 1972, wrote the WHO publication, *Legislative Action to Combat the World Tobacco Epidemic*.[16] In it, she examined how legislation was already being used against the tobacco industry, both to reduce its use and to pave the way toward a society where the product didn't exist at all. These legal strategies had come about in conjunction with the public's growing understanding of the harm caused by secondhand smoke, the nascent world of smokers' rights, and the conviction that the tobacco industry had been getting away with far too much for far too long.

In 1993, at our all-Africa conference on tobacco control in Harare, I had exulted when Roemer openly called for an international treaty approach to tobacco. But for a long while, there was nothing. The movement came to a lumbering, disappointing halt, stymied by Big Tobacco, politicians from WHO's member countries who wanted nothing to do with the idea, and a WHO executive that, for the most part, did not want to rock the boat.

Then, Nakajima decided not to run for a third term and everything changed.

■

In January 1998, the executive board of WHO nominated Dr. Gro Harlem Brundtland[17] as its new director-general, a decision the World Health Assembly supported when its members elected her to the position the following May. In her acceptance speech, she said the organization's key mission was to be the moral voice and technical leader in improving the health of the people of the world, ready and able to give advice that encourages development and alleviates suffering.[18]

"I see our purpose to be combating disease and ill-health, promoting sustainable and equitable health systems in all countries," she said.[19]

Brundtland was someone after my own heart. A former prime minister of Norway and a medical doctor, her sense of global awareness and responsibility began when she was a child who yearned to become a doctor, like her father. He specialized in rehabilitation medicine and won a Rockefeller Foundation scholarship, moving his family to the United States to further his studies. And she had followed in his footsteps, even winning a postdoctoral scholarship to study at Harvard University's School of Public Health, where she learned to look beyond medicine's treatment of symptoms into environmental issues, human development, and the importance of prevention.

"Yes," she said, at her first news conference, "yes, there will be change. A change in focus. A change in the way we organize our work. A change in the way we do things. A change in the way we work as a team."[20]

In December 1983, Javier Pérez de Cuéllar, then UN secretary-general, appointed her to head the World Commission on Environment and Development. The commission's report, *Our Common Future*, was released four years later and would go on to win a highly respected Grawemeyer Award from the University of Louisville for its incisive look at what we are doing to our natural resources and what we can do about it. The awards, established in the mid-1980s by H. Charles Grawemeyer, an industrialist and philanthropist, honor powerful ideas rather than personal achievement. Recipients have included Mikhail Gorbachev, former president of the Soviet

Union; psychiatrist Aaron Beck, regarded as the founder of cognitive therapy; and Linda Darling-Hammond, the Charles E. Ducommun Professor of Education at the Stanford Graduate School of Education, whose work has focused on school restructuring, teacher education, and educational equity.

Taciturn, blunt, and science-oriented, Brundtland was the consummate politician, with a predilection for having all the evidence before making a decision, and the skill for thinking three steps ahead of everyone else. She came into the office with a massive agenda to clean up the organization and make it more focused and relevant again. What, then, would be the hallmarks of her tenure? To help her decide, in the six months between the announcement and her taking the WHO helm in July, she assembled a transition team—and invited me to join it. All of us had one thing in common: we'd been aching to bring about change.

At first, we combed through all the data for both infectious and noncommunicable diseases. When the evidence showed that WHO was neglecting chronic diseases, with a stroke of a pen she changed everything. She put tobacco on the agenda as one of her two big "pathfinder" or legacy projects. The other was called "Rollback Malaria" and was meant to address the particular needs on the African continent. It was exciting that Brundtland chose tobacco control to be the vanguard for non-communicable diseases around the world. Countries sat up and paid attention when she made it as important as a disease that had infected millions.

Brundtland knew that tobacco control was a primary concern in countries that were members of the Organisation for Economic Co-operation and Development and in China, and she knew that to effect the change she wanted, she would have to engage the heads of state, not their health ministers. In one address after her election, she said: "I am a doctor. I believe in science and evidence. Let me state here today: Tobacco is a killer. We need a broad alliance against tobacco, calling on a wide range of partners to halt the relentless increase in global tobacco consumption."[21]

She would make me a key part of that team.

Although it would be a few months before Brundtland anointed me as director of the Tobacco Free Initiative, I hit the ground running, and was already working hard to help frame our strategy. To that end, I'd outlined a proposal for two related initiatives with straightforward titles. "Tobacco Kills—Don't be Duped" would be a two-year international collaboration between media, nongovernmental organizations (NGOs), and experts to spread information about tobacco-related topics, from advertising and sponsorships to advice on how tobacco farmers could diversify into other crops.[22]

The second initiative, "Channeling the Outrage," would lead to the formation in 1999 of the Framework Convention Alliance on Tobacco Control, a confederation of nearly 500 organizations from more than 100 countries that came together to support the talks about tobacco control and to make the ratification and eventual implementation of the treaty a more transparent process.[23]

▪

By September 1998, I was in Washington, DC, making the case for funding these initiatives from an arm's-length foundation that had been specially set up to channel a $1-billion gift that media mogul Ted Turner had given to the United Naitons.

Afterwards, I returned to the hotel room where, jetlagged, I found myself tossing and turning until 3 a.m. Finally, frustrated, I switched on the TV, which was already tuned to CSPAN, the public service network with 24-hour news coverage. Within minutes, I was riveted.

On the screen was a slight, fast-talking guy named Michael Ciresi, who was counsel to the State of Minnesota and Blue Cross and Blue Shield of Minnesota in a lawsuit against Big Tobacco. Unlike other states, which had also filed lawsuits, Ciresi saw the need to go beyond the health consequences and costs of tobacco-related diseases built around the tragic cases of those who had used tobacco and developed cancer. Instead, he filed a RICO case, based on the *Racketeer Influenced and Corrupt Organizations Act*. The case charged that the industry had engaged in a forty-year conspiracy to suppress the health hazards of smoking, had manipulated the nicotine content of cigarettes to keep smokers hooked, and marketed to teenagers to attract new smokers, who would be theirs for life—or until death did them part. It was brilliant, building a case around collusion. Even better, the settlement, which was about to be formally announced, included a requirement that the tobacco companies make about thirty-five million previously hidden documents available to the public on a specially designated website. The companies couldn't just dump the documents on the site, either—like they did with boxes upon boxes of discovery documents in the court cases. They had to provide internal indexes—a kind of road map to their dark, labyrinthine world—which would make it easier for lawyers in other cases to locate incriminating documents.

Easier for us, too.

By now wide-awake, I thought: *I have to meet this guy, if only to thank him from the bottom of my heart.*

As it turned out, Ciresi was speaking at Johns Hopkins, my alma mater, later that very morning. I called old friends there, secured an invitation for lunch, and sped off to meet my new hero. He was slim, with a receding hairline and a wide smile that I imagined was projecting glee at the tobacco decision.

"Sure, we can help," he said. "Meet the 'Document Diva.'"

The diva was Roberta Walburn, the lawyer who headed the effort to actually unearth the secret tobacco papers, a no-nonsense woman who patiently combed through the reams and boxes of discovery material the tobacco companies had sent over in hopes of snowing the legal team under an impenetrable pile of paper. She proved them wrong. Within a few months, she was seconded to Geneva, where, for a year, she helped guide our search through the material and advised us on our plan of attack.

Back at WHO, combing through the documents morning, noon, and night, I grew increasingly scared and disgusted by what I found. It only took a couple of weeks to unearth letters and copies of cheques that proved tobacco companies had bribed ministers of health in a number of countries to corral any attempts at an advertising ban. Academics were paid off, too, including Roger Scruton, a British philosopher and darling of the right wing who, according to *The Guardian*, failed to disclose that Japan Tobacco Inc. was paying him a £4,500 monthly retainer in return for writing opinion pieces in major newspapers that defended the right to smoke. The payments came to light through a series of e-mails in which he asked the company for a £1,000 monthly increase, which would make his take-home pay a tidy £66,000 a year!

I keyed in my own name to discover e-mails that went all the way back to my time at the SAMRC in South Africa. I keyed "Brundtland" into the search engine, too, and my blood went cold. One internal briefing document referred to a speech she had given in 1983 to the Norwegian Society of Cardiology, and stated that she could be "dangerous" if she ever went global. And when she did take the top job at WHO, Philip Morris secretly circulated a document within the industry that read, in part: "Whatever else happens, the election of Brundtland has caused the tobacco issue to be suddenly and dramatically pushed to the top of WHO's action agenda. It is also clear that the new Director-General will be a figure to be reckoned with, that she will bring unusual energy to the fight, and that she has staked much on the outcome."[24]

In other words, Big Tobacco was spoiling for a big battle.

As I printed out that document and a bunch of others, I stared at my phone, sitting mute on my desk. Thoughts were going through my head almost faster than I could process them. Could we be bugged? I wondered.

And: Would tobacco companies stoop that low?

And: Don't pick up the receiver!

Instead, documents in hand, I sprinted up two flights of stairs to Brundtland's office, which was on the seventh floor of WHO headquarters. She was inside, standing with second-in-command Jonas Gahr Støre (who would go on to serve in the Norwegian government and lead the country's Labour Party). At first, she looked concerned at my disheveled appearance and panicked expression. Urgently, I gestured for her to step into the corridor.

"What's wrong?" she asked.

"Ssh," I whispered, putting an index finger to my lips. "I need to speak with you about these documents, but not in your office. You need to see them."

She and Støre came, a bit disbelieving, glancing sidelong at each other. Had I gone squirrely from all the hours I had spent online poring over the documents? But they stood with me in that corridor with its black tiled floor and artifacts on the walls, and the first thing I showed them was the Philip

Morris letter about her. There were other documents, too, about me, about the science and marketing and lies. I showed documents from a conference in Boca Raton in the 1970s, when the heads of the tobacco industry met and decided they needed a strategy—what they called an action plan—to forge policy at WHO and control our work.

"What happened to that action plan?" I asked. "This is serious. These documents prove the tobacco companies have been lying, colluding, paying off people, and undermining our position from the get-go!"

"What should we do?" she wondered, shocked. "How do we respond?"

I had the answer at the ready. "Pull together an independent group of experts and lawyers," I said. "Have them look at how the industry has subverted WHO policies over the years."

"If you need it, we'll do it," she said. "But how?"

At the time, the United Nations had never conducted an inquiry into itself, or even tried. But Brundtland was angry and game. The World Bank should be involved, she decided, so that the inquiry would appear to be at arm's length from WHO. The three other independent commissioners appointed were Dr. David Kessler, then head of the US Food and Drug Administration (FDA); Anke Martiny of Transparency International's branch in Germany; and Thomas Zeltner, a lawyer and doctor and head of the Swiss National Health Authority, who also chaired the inquiry.

It would take about six months for them to investigate and produce their report.[25] We only got to see the edited, sanitized version, with some names and facts blacked out because they were thought to be libellous. Still, they found what we had expected them to: there had been an organized and well-financed effort on the part of the tobacco companies to subvert public policy and impede WHO from carrying out its mission. Their campaigns skirted around the merits of public health issues that surrounded the use of tobacco. Instead, they attempted to divert attention away from health concerns altogether and distort the results of scientific studies. They tried to reduce the funding allocated to WHO's scientific and policy initiatives, to pit other UN agencies against the organization, and to convince officials and politicians in developing countries that WHO wanted to implement a First World agenda at the expense of their own Third World populations.

We were going to stop them.

4

TAKING ON BIG TOBACCO

From military bosses to police officers, from the reporter who couldn't believe I'd legitimately lost a swimming race to a Coloured man to Rembrandt boss Anton Rupert and his son Johann, I'd spent much of my life standing up, with varying degrees of success, to people who were stuck in their way of thinking for a variety of reasons, from money to ignorance and institutionalized racism. In July 1998, as we officially launched the Tobacco Free Initiative that would lead to the signing of the Framework Convention on Tobacco Control five years later, it felt like I—like *we*—were finally on the road to making a difference at the global level. If I couldn't dislodge the Ruperts of the world from their way of thinking, I could at least change the way people thought about *them*. I couldn't

imagine a better time to be involved in a project of this mag-
nitude. We saw it as the good fight: good knights against evil
tobacco. I was tagged to lead the initiative.

Brundtland had done her homework, consulting with
tobacco experts such as Sir Richard Peto, a professor in the
medical school at Oxford University, and demographer Alan
Lopez, co-author (with Christopher Murray) of the seminal
Global Burden of Disease assessment. Since its release in 1996,
this study has played a key role in how government and WHO
set their health priorities and allocate resources.[26] In addition,
in the early 1990s, Lopez and Peto had worked together on
another publication, the "Peto-Lopez Method," a formula that
estimates the number of deaths due to tobacco-related causes
and helps support the policy decisions of health professionals
and governments.[27]

With all that in mind, the first order of business was to
prepare a preliminary report that outlined the steps we would
have to take in order to establish our mission. The big picture
goals were, first, to determine the burden of disease on governments and health care systems, what the trends were, and
what, if anything, was preventable. Second, we had to build a
team to drive change and address a global health threat, and
to shine a bright light on the tobacco industry's role over the
years, over the decades, over nearly *half a century* to thwart
science and progress.

After we gave Brundtland the report, she called us to her
office for a meeting. It didn't last long. She heard us out, then

said, simply: "Go away. Take some time to figure out how much money you need and come back with an initial plan."

It took Bettcher and me just over a month. He had been at my side since we worked on the "Health for All in the 21st Century" report (and has since become director of WHO's Department for Prevention of Noncommunicable Diseases). We soon knew we weren't going to ask for funding to cover the next six months or even the next six years. We weren't going that small. We were setting our sights much higher, asking for a whole future: this meant a large amount of money to carry us years and years down the road.

"Douglas, forget our policy work, plodding from one day to the next," I said. "That ends now. From now on, we're planning a global tobacco program."

We wanted an international tobacco control treaty between the then-192 member countries of WHO—the first treaty in the world to be entirely devoted to a public health issue. The kind of treaty that Allyn Taylor first wrote about in the *American Journal of Law and Medicine* and that Roemer had called for from the podium in Harare. That's what we went and told Brundtland.

Were we nervous? Maybe a bit. But in South Africa, I had learned to ask for the moon and if I didn't always get it, then I'd find another way. And, as we noted, if we didn't ask, then we'd never know what we could have gotten in the first place.

Brundtland grilled us up, down, and sideways to make sure we had properly mapped out what we wanted to do and taken into account the possible pitfalls and booby traps. Then she gave us what we asked for. We were thrilled at our good fortune. This was political support like we had never had before, and all on a topic that the previous executive had no interest in. As long as we could make a good case, we knew she would support our efforts and shield us from those who would do anything to see us fail.

To help us spin our tobacco story—the *true* tobacco story—Brundtland brought in Chitra Subramaniam to take charge of media relations. Brundtland knew Chitra, as everyone called her, because she had helped with Brundtland's campaign to become director-general. A former UN correspondent based in Geneva, Chitra's 1987 story about Swedish arms manufacturer Bofors paying illegal kickbacks to Swedish and Indian politicians in connection with a $1.4-billion sale of the company's field howitzers to India had exposed corruption at the highest levels. Heavily pregnant at the time, she was fearless in the face of threats. Rajiv Gandhi, then prime minister of India, contemptuously called her a "girl reporter,"[28] yet because of the scandal, his government fell in the general election of 1989.

Brundtland figured the former journalist would be perfect for the job—calm, strong, and commonsensical in the face of international protest, be it at the instigation of tobacco companies or not. She would see a way to turn the tables on the companies by shifting the debate away from their self-serving, long-standing justification for their existence, which went something like this: Smoking was a choice and an activity you could turn on and off at will. If you wanted to stop and couldn't, it was your problem not the companies'. They simply made something that people enjoyed, and they supported causes and organizations that contributed to culture and other integral facets of society.

I'd first heard a version of this argument when I was a determined, naive medical student in Anton Rupert's boardroom at Rembrandt all those years ago. I could have used Chitra then—and I was grateful for her presence now.

With her help, we were able to reframe the debate, from one focused on individual choice and what many health officials considered to be people who simply lacked willpower to one that addressed tobacco companies' corporate abuses and lack of accountability. Bolstered by the disclosure of incriminating documents on the website that the tobacco companies were ordered to build as part of the Minnesota court settlement, we had a good case. Actually, we had a great case, complete with evidence showing the depths to which the companies had sunk to suppress or slow down research. We could prove beyond any doubt that Big Tobacco had worked to keep tobacco control off the agenda of major national and international health organizations. We could also guarantee that their techniques wouldn't work any longer, because we could monitor their actions through the documents.

There were no more secrets, even if the tobacco companies kept trying. An undated BAT document titled "The World

Health Organization and the Tobacco Free Initiative" was about how to stop us altogether. Russia, it said, is a member of WHO's executive board, and with that country as an ally, an "interagency taskforce" had been established to "deal with the WHO TFI" and to "combat it." The way forward, it said, was threefold: lobby finance, tax, and agriculture ministries around the world; keep the convention as broadly worded as possible; and slow the process down on the grounds that more internal consultation was needed.

Notes for a speech Martin Broughton, chair of BAT, gave at the World Economic Forum in January 1999, perfectly encapsulated the industry position. "Let's face it, living is risky," they read. "We can only live once—let's enjoy it while we can." The notes continued that we at the Tobacco Free Initiative, driven by Western idealism, were overreacting, spending our time trying to eliminate smoking rather than tackling "real issues" in the developing world such as malnutrition, sanitation, and infant mortality.[29]

At every turn, judging by the notes, the companies tried to undermine my credibility and that of WHO in general. Why weren't we concentrating on measles and immunization campaigns? Why wouldn't we stick to issues that really mattered, namely, communicable diseases? Why did we have to tackle tobacco products, which they claimed consumers *loved*?

Yasmin, who was observing the drama from the sidelines, was more scared for my professional future than I was. I was focused strictly on the issues, and it felt like there wasn't a time we weren't working, wading through papers and arguments. Nights, weekends, online, and on the phone, speaking with the people working with us in places like Zimbabwe, Malawi, and India, with medical experts, and with representatives from cultural organizations. When tobacco farmers cried that their livelihoods would be destroyed, we tried to assuage them, told them their fears were misplaced. It would be decades before they saw even a bit of impact, because no matter our intentions, no matter that the name of the division I headed contained the phrase "tobacco-free," we didn't envision a world completely without tobacco. Taxes would still be considerable, as would the demand for raw product.

Really, we just wanted to reduce tobacco consumption and ensure people were making informed decisions when they decided to light up. And while the epidemiological data on death was crucial for us, we found that it was the financial data—the cost of health care and unemployment benefits and the loss of work hours due to smoking-relating illnesses—that made politicians reconsider their opposition to us.

■

In all, the process took five years—the whole of Brundtland's term in office. We knew she might not run a second time, so if we didn't finish negotiations and get the treaty signed before May 2003, we risked losing it all. All the work. All the capital.

Everything. We knew the next director-general would have his or her own agenda, and this initiative was not universally popular in the organization. Nor was it cheap. Imagine: each time we convened a meeting to negotiate, it cost WHO about $1 million because we had to pay for the travel and accommodation of the representatives of every country involved.

During the process, we invited tobacco companies to take part on two fronts. Hoping that we could locate some kind of nexus where we could work together, the first front was the creation of what we called the Tobacco Regulation Committee. We invited researchers and scientists from all the companies to come talk, to explain to us what their science was all about. It marked the first time I heard about the concept of harm reduction, of products the companies were working on to reduce the risk of contracting a tobacco-related disease. But it was hard to take them seriously, because their presentations were sloppy and insubstantial—mostly, if not entirely, spin. Their scientists did not speak to us. Their public relations representatives did. Dr. Chris Proctor of BAT, ostensibly a scientist, was commanded to use the company's public relations line by Fran Morrison, the formidable head of corporate communication and a pro-smoking stalwart. From the website documents, I knew that Proctor had reported on me and my background to his superiors.

At the end of the process, it was clear that the committee had done nothing for either side, save to reinforce that the companies still believed, or hoped, the process wouldn't go anywhere.

The second front was two days of public hearings in the spring of 1999, where any legitimate party with a stake in the matter—NGOs, tobacco companies, and even the Association of Hemp Growers, which complained that WHO was giving their crop a bad rap—could speak. It was a bit of a circus, to say the least, raucous and overflowing. Each tobacco company made sure their representatives were at each hearing so that for the outside world they could spin whatever happened that day in their favor. For the most part, they were intent—and very stressed. One lasting image I have is of David Davies, an executive at PMI, sitting there sweating, with bloodstains on his shirt. He'd cut himself shaving that morning and was so rushed, he didn't even notice!

Only one of the tobacco people—a lawyer who at the time was employed by BAT—made a genuine effort to understand what was going on and what the real issues were. Although she was a "spy," I liked and respected her. Elegant and straight talking, with a passion for whiskey, cigars, shoes, and women's health, her central focus at the hearings was the illicit trade in tobacco. A few years down the road, it would be an e-mail from her that would turn my career in a different direction.

Next up was a series of high-level meetings that required a new infrastructure, because it was the first time WHO had to convene government representatives on a regular basis to discuss only one topic. They were held in a conference center that had been built in Geneva during the Cold War, complete with sliding-panel walls (to avoid someone you didn't want to speak to), concealed corridors, and hidden offices. Each session would last seven to ten days, and the WHO staff had to tread lightly: governments were supposed to be the activists here, not us.

Instead, we worked in the background, researching candidates who could chair the meetings, who knew how to negotiate political treaties—an ambassador living in Geneva who could represent a country with an interest in the tobacco industry, be it farming or production. We fixed on Celso Luiz Nunes Amorim of Brazil, a country that was starting to show an interest in the rates of tobacco consumption and was reputed to have skilled foreign policy people who were incorruptible.

Brundtland and I had dinner with Amorim and his wife at the Brazilian embassy. When she asked if he would stand for election by his peers to become chairman, he said yes, except there was one big problem: "I smoke."

His wife leaned over. "Well," she said, "it's a good reason for you to quit, isn't it?"

To his credit, he did.

Other ambassadors tried to subvert or at least slow down the process. One evening, Brundtland and I were invited to dine with the Turkish ambassador. I was seated next to his trade representative, a fast-talking young woman who had evidently been instructed to persuade me we didn't need a treaty at all. Yet there was nary a mention throughout the meal of Turkey's close relationship with BAT, of which we were very well aware. At the end of the evening, the ambassador asked if our minds had been changed.

"No," Brundtland said. "I'm convinced we need it more than ever."

The pressure wouldn't stop. Martin Broughton of BAT, who spoke so menacingly at the World Economic Forum back in 1999, indicated that his company would voluntarily work with others to tighten up access to tobacco, among other things; therefore, there was no need for a binding treaty. Later, in a letter to Brundtland that was publicized in the media, the company suggested that WHO wasn't willing to negotiate with industry. It was ironic, given that we had invited the industry to participate. We wanted them to negotiate.

In late December 1998, the industry lit on the idea to have a private debate in Davos, Switzerland, about the treaty, with Broughton, a representative from the American Civil Liberties Union (ACLU), and me. Walburn, the Document Diva from Minnesota, worked hard to prepare me. I walked into the room, which was filled with about seventy people. The first person I saw was Ken Clarke, the deputy head of the British Conservative Party, a pro-tobacco advocate who sat on BAT's board and had been appointed health minister in 1988. On his lap was a fluffy little brown dog, and his wife sat next to him, knitting.

I must say, it was a strange scene.

The ACLU representative was ready to start things off by saying this was a case that revolved around freedom of choice. I was ready for that, and before the debate even began, I took her aside.

"Let's come to an agreement," I said. "We found a letter among the tobacco documents online referring to a million-dollar contract between Philip Morris and the ACLU ensuring that freedom of choice is addressed in the tobacco debate. Basically, you were bought off and if you start making arguments about choice, I'll be forced to read this letter out loud."

When the debate started, she didn't say anything of substance. To this day, I don't think many people know about the letter. But they should.

■

For over three years, we worked and sweated. In that time, there were multiple meetings that lasted up to ten days at a time and involved hundreds of representatives from countries around the world. Mostly, we met in the large committee room at the Geneva International Conference Centre, a space that can accommodate up to 2,200. But there were lots of smaller breakaway meetings, too, as people argued over the wording to a paragraph or the perceived sense of a clause. It marked the first time that WHO paid for people to travel to Geneva for just one specific purpose—to hammer out a treaty on tobacco control—rather than to attend a series of meetings that involved the organization's various departments. And even though the topic itself was touchy, the mood was polite, even sedate. When people wanted to speak, they would hold up a placard. Messengers drifted around the room, delivering missives and requests, and the galleries were full of observers who represented any number of NGOs and other groups who'd signed up to witness the laborious process of history being made.

As we neared the end of our three-year process, we shifted into high gear. In a mad scramble, for days and nights on end in a cavernous room in Geneva's Palais des Nations, over five hundred people hammered out the final points of an agreement in a Babel of languages. At 10 p.m. on February 28, 2003, everyone was so exhausted and strung out that we agreed to take a short break. To go back to our offices, our homes, our embassies for showers and a change of clothes. There were only a few hours left. I rushed back to Échenevex, driving madly on side roads to make it home in fifteen minutes to check in with Yasmin, who was eight months pregnant.

My mind was on the translators. Few others were aware that they had been contracted for only a set period of time and that we would lose them at 4 a.m. And because of their tight schedules, they would not be available again until that May. We were so close! But Brundtland, ever the pragmatic politician, had decreed that nothing is agreed until everything is agreed, and if the translators were gone, then we were finished. Everything we'd worked for—from advertising bans and higher excise taxes to limits on lobbying, a restriction on sales to minors, and protection from secondhand smoke— would be up in smoke! By now, I had an inkling that Brundt- land would not stand for reelection as director-general—and who knew if her successor would have the same priorities.

I thought: *You're a swimmer. You see the end. You go for it, no matter how you're feeling.*

My cell phone rang. It was the German ambassador.

"We're very happy with the treaty," he began. "We just want to add a reservation clause at the end that says we agree to everything but reserve the right not to agree."

I froze. Clauses like that are often put in parts of a treaty to coax a final country to sign, but I knew if this was raised on the floor, we were in big trouble because the European Union would be voting as a bloc. If one dissented, they all would.

"I'll call the director-general," I said. "Let me get back to you."

My conversation with Brundtland lasted all of ten seconds. "No," she said.

I relayed her answer to the German ambassador, and returned to the negotiations wondering if it all had been for naught. Five years of research, travel, and strong-arming, of trying to finish something I had longed to do ever since I was a medical student. And now I had no idea what Ger- many was going to do. For that matter, I didn't even know what the United States was going to do, given that the Bush administration didn't like the idea of the treaty one bit. But the United Stated didn't have to agree. For them, because of their role at the United Nations, ratification would be a two-step process. Having the United States abstain or vote "no" wouldn't be the end of the world. But oh my God, if we lost the translators ...

We convened again just after midnight. Tommy Thompson, US secretary for health and human services, came to that final round and supported the treaty. We were amazed when he said it was good for public health. The European delegate spoke for all of the European Union, and there was not a peep from the German.

An hour later, translators still in place, we had a deal in principle.

And May 21, 2003, at the 56th World Health Assembly in Geneva, *192* countries unanimously voted to become signatories to it.[30] Yasmin and I were in attendance, as was our son, Julian, born on April 18, a birthday he almost shares with Brundtland's own two days later. He was a cooing, uncranky witness to history.

That day, I felt on top of the world. It didn't matter that with a new director-general about to take over from Brundtland, my future at WHO was uncertain. My team and I had made a difference, and on that day, it was enough.

But the feeling wouldn't last long. Changes were coming.

5

THE END
OF THE
BEGINNING

After the tobacco control treaty was signed, it would have been nice to have some time to catch my breath, to spend time with Yasmin and our newborn son. Instead, I found myself caught up once again in a huge project—one that had begun in 2002, even as the tobacco negotiations continued.

It was a dizzyingly busy time. As of 2002, the Tobacco Free Initiative was not my only responsibility since Brundtland had appointed me the head of all noncommunicable disease divisions at WHO, including obesity and type 2 diabetes. In a speech to health ministers at WHO's annual general meeting that year in London, she named obesity, high blood pressure, and unhealthy cholesterol levels as the next big, bad problems she wanted the organization to take on. In other words, she was putting the food industry on notice: after the tobacco treaty was completed, WHO was coming after companies that produced high-fat, high-sugar, high-salt products. Questions—actually the same question, in different forms—began coming at me, over and over, from beer makers, potato chip manufacturers, and media outlets such as the *New York Times*:

"After tobacco, are we next?"

"Is WHO coming for us?"

"Are you going to try for a treaty that regulates food industries, too?"

I didn't know how to respond. "Yes, sort of" would have been accurate. As would have "No, not really."

The first challenge was that we had no means of talking to the food industry. WHO didn't have a marketing arm or similar structure in place to address the concerns and fears being expressed, nor was there a separate entity that represented the interests of the food industry. Our own lawyers would have been horrified at the notion of us approaching the industry directly with no strategy in place. Doing so could have been seen as an attempt to create policy while in cahoots with the very companies we wanted to regulate.

To bridge the gap, we hired two consultants with long histories working with big business and government, Robert Davies and Harriet Mouchly-Weiss. Davies was the brilliant, dedicated chief executive of the Prince of Wales International Business Leaders Forum, a man who had spent his entire career trying to harness the power and creativity of private enterprise to the vision and values of the public sector. He was the yin to Mouchly-Weiss's yang: she was a diminutive, gray-haired force of nature who had built a career as a key advisor to heads of government and CEOs of Fortune 500 companies. When they spoke, we listened. When they advised, we took heed. And when Mouchly-Weiss told me that no matter what our lawyers thought, I was going to have dinner with Niels Christiansen, head of nutrition and public relations at Nestlé S.A., one of her former clients, to wrestle out our differences, I meekly asked: "What night and time?" I never told her of the image that came to mind, me facing an opponent across a table, our shirtsleeves rolled up, grimacing as we arm-wrestled.

What would I have to say to someone whose company made Smarties and Nesquik Milk Chocolatey Cereal, and, worst of all, marketed its infant formula in developing countries where, mixed with contaminated water, it caused diarrhea and led to many infant fatalities. That debacle had resulted in a years-long international boycott of Nestlé products, and the company still remained defensive and tight-lipped about it. How would it even be possible to have a frank and honest discussion with Nestlé about obesity and all it entailed?

But if Mouchly-Weiss wanted it, I was willing to listen. And I knew this was a good way to be heard.

That's how, on a chilly autumn evening in 2002, I found myself standing outside the restaurant-bar L'Orangerie on Boulevard Helvétique in a tranquil corner of Geneva. I wondered if Christiansen had chosen it because it was far from both our places of work, with less chance of people we each worked with seeing us together.

I thought: *Harriet will kill me if I don't go in. Besides, when did I ever refuse to listen to the other side? Remember Rembrandt!*

Taking a deep breath, I pulled open the restaurant's heavy main door and walked in. The first thing I noticed was the subdued lighting, thick stone walls, and tables spaced far enough apart to have a conversation with no neighboring diner listening in. Christiansen, tall, with white hair swept back off his forehead and a neat white goatee, was waiting with a large gift box, which he handed to me—After Eight chocolate mints, which I adore. (At the time, I had no idea they were made by Nestlé; as far as "bribes" went, the only thing I would ever inadvertently count would be calories.) He'd done his research—or Mouchly-Weiss had done it for him, as she had done for me.

"Don't leave anything to chance" was her watchword and modus operandi.

I thanked Christiansen, and sat down.

We spent over two hours together, lingering over chocolate mousse and espressos, laying out our cases and concerns, back and forth and much franker than I had thought possible.

Thank you, Harriet.

As a public health expert, I often thought of food companies as a bane, purveyors of too much salt, sugar, and fat, of potato chips, soft drinks, processed cheese, chemically cured cold cuts, and candy. To the food companies, WHO was like a finger-pointing parent who always thought it knew better and wanted to ground them—or erase them from existence altogether.

Christiansen, who began working at Nestlé long after the infant formula debacle began, said Brundtland's speech at WHO's annual meeting didn't help matters.

"It sounds like you're coming for us," he continued. "Are you?"

There it was again—the question!

"No, not exactly," I said. From my experience as an epidemiologist in South Africa and at WHO, I didn't think something similar to the tobacco control treaty was the way to go in this case, I explained. The issues surrounding food consumption and physical activity were as different from tobacco as white is to black. Sugar wasn't the new tobacco. Neither was salt nor fat. I already knew that. With tobacco, the only players on the international stage were four multinational companies (and the Chinese government, which held the monopoly in that country). As we would outline in a paper already submitted to the *Journal of Public Health Policy*, which would be published the following year, with years of data to back us up, we could demonstrate a *direct* link between tobacco use, disease, and death.[31]

The same could not be said about nutrition, which was made up of myriad players and products. We weren't going to turn junk food into the new tobacco. There was no way to ban or control the consumption of hamburgers in public places. Ditto for chips, chocolate cereal, soda, or, come to think of it, After Eight mints.

I said all this to Christiansen, then asked: "Are there areas we could agree to change marketing on, on a global basis? Is there an answer that is plain old common sense?"

To my pleasant surprise, he agreed that the fight against obesity required more than simply telling people to get off their butts and do more exercise. Instead, it needed governments, public health organizations, and private enterprise to somehow work together to drive the message home: eating more healthfully and getting out to do anything—a jog, a hike up a mountain, a bike ride along a lake, or simply walking the dog—led to a longer and better quality of life.

Painstakingly, he laid out the concerns of shareholders and marketers. What would happen to profit and growth? There were commodity prices to consider and the high cost of research and development. What could he say to his bosses that would ease their minds?

I wasn't sure. I wish I *could* have told him something that would make the company feel better. Nevertheless, at the end of the dinner, as we scooped the last of the chocolate mousse, we at least agreed we had enough in common to convene a series of preparatory policy development meetings between WHO and a range of companies such as Nestlé and Unilever, with the final goal of having Brundtland meet with the CEOs in a summit at a location to be determined.

We knew there would be roadblocks along the way, among them getting NGOs to come on board to help push an agreement forward. Many were already critical of many of the big food companies in general, so Christiansen and I both knew they would be especially horrified at the idea of working in concert with Nestlé, the company they called a "baby killer."

"But if we don't try, we'll never know," I said. "Nothing ventured, nothing gained."

"You're right," he replied. We shook on it, promising to speak soon.

I liked his professionalism and his realistic approach to change. If we could get along—two people who worked for organizations that were bitter enemies—maybe, just maybe we could bring other "resisters" into the circle.

It was a start.

■

Throughout my career, one of my heroes has been Dr. Charles-Edward Amory Winslow, the founder of the public health program at Yale University in the early 1900s. He was a man who thought not only outside but also far beyond the box, calling for the medical community to rise above an ambulance-like tendency to focus on and treat only what was directly in front of it. "Redefine the unacceptable" was his war cry. Take on the unthinkable. Be open to changing your mind because public health itself is not a static discipline but, rather, a social science. Observers and movers, we should push the field in new directions and use whatever tools were at our disposal, no matter how conventional or not. The end goals were always changing. It could be potable water and food free of pesticides, or housing that was ventilated, heated, and pest-free, or a safe workplace. I had followed those principles while running the Tobacco Free Initiative, and now, I meant to put them to use in a different arena.

As a member of the WHO committee drafting new dietary guidelines, I needed to look at the big picture of food, too. The draft would be circulated among WHO's member states and multinational companies for discussion, and for the first time in WHO's history, it would be on the Internet, inviting comments from anybody who had something to say, be it a top medical researcher at the Karolinska Institutet in Sweden or Joe Blow from proverbial Podunk, USA. The point was to be as transparent as possible. We called it a "Global Strategy on Diet, Physical Activity and Health."[32] There was not even a hint of the word "treaty." This time, it *was* different.

Although the recommendations contained in the draft seemed modest, and made perfect sense to nutritionists and other public health professionals who saw the toll taken by obesity and type 2 diabetes around the world, some of our strategy caused controversy. Actually, controversy is probably a massive understatement. Basically, all hell broke loose. The food industry was in an uproar, upset that the working paper had been posted in a public domain where anyone could see our suggestions on dietary change. Suggestions such as people limiting their salt intake to 5 grams a day and their sugar consumption to 10 per cent of their total daily calories. Previously disparate lobby groups for salt, palm oil, and sugar had united to pressure WHO to reverse its positions. We were seen as anti-business, anti-soda, and anti–junk food. We were "wonky scientists" up against a trillion-dollar industry that had powerful lobbies and government contacts around the world.

The United States Cattlemen's Association vehemently opposed a proposal that people eat less red meat. And the palm oil industry—an environmental disaster already, with carbon-conserving tropical rainforests plowed over to make way for monoculture plantations and the burning of fossil fuels—was furious that we said the product may increase one's chance of developing heart disease—which it does. I'll never forget the Malaysian ambassador to the United Nations storming into a meeting she'd demanded with Brundtland and me, asking why we wanted to destroy the social and economic underpinnings of her country and others that depended on the profit generated by palm oil.

"If you insist on going ahead, then Malaysia will form a common front with Indonesia and Saudi Arabia and charge that WHO is mounting an attack on leading Muslim countries," she said.

It was a clear threat, but Brundtland did not budge. To this day, I believe the palm oil lobby is just as, if not more, guilty of subverting public health policy than the tobacco companies ever were. Only environmental groups such as Greenpeace have ever made a point of talking about it.

But of them all, the sugar industry was the most vehement. Under the auspices of the International Sugar Association, which bills itself as the "scientific voice" of the industry in the United States, it wrote a blistering letter to Brundtland that threatened to "exercise every avenue available to expose the dubious nature" of the report. "Taxpayers' dollars should not be used to support misguided, non-science-based reports which do not add to the health and well-being of Americans, much less the rest of the world," it read. "If necessary we will promote and encourage new laws which require future WHO funding to be provided only if the organisation accepts that all reports must be supported by the preponderance of science."[33]

It pressured Tommy Thompson, US health secretary, to punish WHO by cutting off the $406 million in funds it transferred annually to the organization until we came to our senses. And it was supported by two senators, John Breaux of Louisiana and Larry Craig from Idaho, who happened to be co-chairs of the US Senate Sweetener Caucus, and by six other big American food organizations, including the United States Council for International Business, a coalition of companies that counted among its members major players such as Coca-Cola and PepsiCo. They all claimed that our research, which was based on the work of thirty health and nutrition experts after consulting with another thirty internationally respected scientists around the world, was fundamentally and scientifically flawed. This, they said, was because the health and medicine division of the US National Academies of Sciences, Engineering, and Medicine had issued a report in 2002 that stated added sugars could amount to as much as 25 per cent of a person's daily diet without harming one's health.[34]

Was I surprised at the intensity of the response? Not really. When we started the initiative, Phil James, president of the International Association for the Study of Obesity and a colleague who'd been involved in a previous report back in the 1990s and who now headed WHO's task force on obesity, took me aside. "Watch out for the sugar industry," he warned me. "Prepare yourself. They'll come after you hard."

A few big companies such as Unilever did respond to the report in positive fashion, accelerating their investments in fruit and vegetable products. I remember representatives coming to visit us at WHO with laboratory-like samples from a new juice line that included a strawberry-kale mixture. But the majority responded with fear and a bully's automatic reflex to push back hard.

The only answer we had was the evidence we presented.

Even as we were beset by aggressive, well-organized producers of unhealthy foods, lobbyists, and screaming government representatives, we were also hampered by the fact that groups that did produce healthy foods tended not to have lobbyists, couldn't organize themselves, and ended up mostly mute in the debate. If they'd been able to be more vocal—to stand up and speak to the benefits of fruits, vegetables, whole grains, and other such products; of cheese that wasn't sickly orange and processed; of meat and fish that weren't pumped full of additives—I'm sure it would have helped. At least, I like to think so.

The one exception was the International Bean Alliance, which capitalized on the fact that we praised all varieties of their low-fat, high-fiber, protein-rich product, save for its unfortunate tendency to cause gas. But you didn't, and still don't, hear banana producers on the stump about the benefits of eating a fruit chock-full of potassium, antioxidants, and fiber, or almond growers or orange producers or fresh vegetable growers.

Still, we didn't give up.

In the midst of all the drama, I quietly continued informal talks with Christiansen and representatives of other multinational companies in an effort to reach some kind of entente and engineer some kind of summit between Brundtland and the CEOs. As was her habit, the director-general did not want to go into a meeting where the outcome was unknown. To do so would risk damaging WHO's image before the world and affect its ability to negotiate in the future. I sent out copies of the draft guidelines and got them back, marked up and annotated.

As it turned out, our last such informal talk was held in March 2003, a round table at a lovely little inn, the Auberge des Chasseurs in sleepy Échenevex, France. Yasmin and I had moved there after years in Nyon because we needed more space with a baby on the way. We were under pressure to arrange a summit the following month, before Brundtland announced at WHO's annual general meeting in May that she would be leaving her post at the end of August. The unknown was already looming ahead of us: who knew who would replace her or what the new leadership's priorities would be. We wanted to get the draft guidelines in for an agreement before we had to face that eventuality.

Located about 12.5 miles from Geneva, Échenevex is a village of just over 1,400 inhabitants, with a man-made beach. At the time we met, fields were freshly sown with wheat and sunflowers were already in bloom along the banks of a slow-moving stream.

Bring them to my home ground, I thought. The auberge was more welcoming and secure than a cold, official meeting room in a WHO building in Geneva, especially for a group that had initially sworn they would never speak to us but had grudgingly come around. We could speak freely here, and if we wanted to yell at each other, we could do so in the great outdoors with only cows chewing their cud to hear us.

The running of the bulls, or, more accurately, the bull-headed, I told myself.

So, unbeknownst to villagers, about twenty executives from a number of Fortune 500 companies began to show up at the auberge, driven in black limousines from the airport or in personal cars from homes in the area. Representatives from Coca-Cola, Texaco, and Danone mingled with those from Unilever, Nestlé, Kraft, Kellogg, and Grupo Bimbo, a Mexican multinational that is the world's largest bakery company.

Leave nothing to chance was our motto, and make sure there is agreement. How could we formulate guidelines that would make the various marketing departments happy? What tools—sweeteners, really—could we write into the draft to make companies willing to abide by the guidelines in the first place? I was aware that some 12-ounce cans of regular soda, for example, contained more than double the daily sugar limit recommended by nutritionists—nine teaspoons for men and six for women.

Somehow, though, there was grudging acceptance, and the summit between Brundtland and the CEOs went ahead that April, the first of what were supposed to be more "scripted" meetings to formulate policy. For the most part, it was a success—and quite civil, to boot, although Brundtland, because of the optics, refused to attend a cocktail party hosted by Coca-Cola. She didn't want to look like a lame duck or a lackey of big business. Neither did we. We had come so far. It was unthinkable that the legacy of the projects she championed would be left hanging.

Alas, further meetings weren't to be.

The guidelines eventually passed, exactly as we wrote them, at the next World Health Assembly in May 2004. However, Brundtland's successor, Lee Jong-wook, a South Korean public health specialist who had risen through WHO's ranks on the infectious diseases side, didn't place much emphasis on them. Earlier that year, he'd received a thirty-page letter from William (Bill) Steiger, at the time US representative to WHO's executive board, complaining that the guidelines didn't meet American standards because they lacked transparency and were not subject to external evaluation or peer review.[35] Having sought expert opinions through consultations and hearings, and having posted the draft guidelines on the Internet for everyone to see and comment on, I would have been puzzled over what he meant if I wasn't aware of industry-dictated pressures.

The guidelines simply and quietly sank out of sight, a casualty of political change, available to those who looked for them on the WHO website. But that was it.

It was not surprising that the departure of Brundtland, as with that of many other directors-general who came before her, heralded a changing of the guard and of priorities. Rare was the new leader who kept the staff who defined the tenure of a predecessor. Lee wanted to bring in his own people, which I understood. He didn't fire me—he couldn't—but he did have the right to remove me from my post. Which he did, shunting me off to what WHO employees all called the "waiting room."

It was the beginning of the end. I was waiting to go. I had just one more thing to do.

6

TREADING WATER

My old office had been the largest and most luxurious
I'd ever had, with three secretaries in the anteroom, space for
ten people to comfortably sit around a table and spread out
papers, and a view of Geneva that I never tired of looking
at. Now, I was moved to a workspace—the infamous waiting room—that was little more than a cubicle, with a simple
desk, two hardback chairs, and a window that looked out on
a very busy parking lot. Located in a covered corridor that
connected the main WHO building to the cafeteria, it was the
middle of nowhere, and a dramatic comedown. Once, I had
been responsible for a staff of 250 people and had the ear of
the director-general. Now, I answered my own phone and had
a staff of exactly one: researcher Corinna Hawkes.

There were black moments, hours, and days. I'd be lying if I said there weren't. But I was confident there would be other job offers. To be sure, I had made enemies in my work, but I also had wonderful networks of friends and professional contacts. I'd learned patience and persistence. As long as I worked hard and bided my time, change would come.

So, every day I made sure to laugh and to swim, fighting the waves in Lake Geneva or doing laps in a pool. Yasmin was my great listener and sounding board, and now we had our son Julian.

Our little family in rural Échenevex had breakfasts and dinners together, and long walks along the lake. In the evenings, we pushed Julian in his pram, pointing out horses and cows. He was such a happy baby, responsive and engaged in what was going on around him. And it was obvious from before he could walk that he loved everything to do with balls, presaging a future as a serious tennis player.

Meanwhile, I undertook the job Lee had given me—to develop and write an international noncommunicable disease strategy—within the timeline he'd set—one year. The strategy was meant to help fulfill a promise Lee made at a news conference when he took office in July 2003: "Noncommunicable diseases and injuries account for a growing share—now about 60 per cent—of the burden of disease worldwide, [so] we will develop and implement a comprehensive plan for fighting [them]."[36] Unspoken in his statement was an acknowledgement that even though WHO had made progress in the fight against such diseases—the tobacco control treaty, for example, and the global strategy on diet, physical activity, and health—it was still unclear how it should respond to such threats in the future in a way that would help its member states and garner their support.

With Corinna Hawkes, who is now the director of the Centre for Food Policy at City, University of London, I started working on what we called "Towards a WHO long-term strategy for prevention and control of leading chronic diseases."[37] We wanted to do the best job possible while not compromising on ideals I held dear and knew were right, even if at the moment the project itself was getting no support from on high—and neither was I.

We put together a steering committee that included Janet Voûte, then CEO of the World Heart Federation, and Dr. Alfredo Morabia, at the time a medical professor at the University of Geneva and now editor of the *American Journal of Public Health*. The committee presented an eighty-six-page rationale for action, conducted a financial and policy review of how key stakeholders—among them G8 countries, UNICEF, and the World Bank—could align their policies to be more supportive of fighting noncommunicable diseases, and made seven central recommendations for both long-term disease prevention and disease control.

We were driven by the fact that mortality and the burden of leading chronic diseases, including cancer and diabetes, was rising over the long term, particularly in developing countries. In India and South Africa, for example, the cardiovascular death rates for women between the ages of 35 and 64 were higher in 2003 than they were for women of the same age range in the United States in the 1950s, when risk levels were higher and medicine less advanced. And we found that over half of the projected *9 million* deaths from cardiovascular disease in China by 2030 will be people in the 35-to-64 age range.

When we looked at foreign investment in developing countries, we found that in 2002 alone, organizations such as WHO, the World Bank, and bilateral development agencies were, at US$69 million, lagging far behind the US$327 million invested by food, beverage, and tobacco concerns. We called for more private and public partnerships, for big business to work in concert with nonprofit and government organizations, because pooling resources in the pursuit of a common goal was the best solution of all.

It felt bittersweet that the strategy would be my final contribution to the organization that had so defined my professional life for the previous nine years. So much had been good about the experience. Brundtland had been a dynamic, committed, no-nonsense director-general, and in working for her, I had been part of a movement that set the pace for change when it came to tobacco and, to a lesser extent, food and physical activity. For that, I was grateful and proud. This strategy would be the final block in my legacy, a compilation of everything I had learned in South Africa and at WHO.

I would leave when it was done, published, and placed in Lee's hands for him to do with what he wanted.

Maybe I naively hoped Lee was serious about using it, or that once he saw what we were doing, he'd realize how important the issues were. But there was no internal institutional support for something like this study—if there had been any in the first place. My only hope was that it could have an impact beyond WHO, and so I started to write an article for the *Journal of the American Medical Association*. Published in 2004, "The Global Burden of Chronic Diseases" is now one of the most cited pieces on the urgent need for action around the world.[38]

■

As we toiled in the bowels of WHO's headquarters, wanting—*determined*—to produce a report that could make a difference, no matter Lee's lack of interest, I met people who brought back memories of a project I first heard about in the mid-1980s, when I was still in South Africa at the SAMRC. The pharmaceutical giant Merck & Company, Inc.—where scientists had invented the mumps and rubella vaccines, where the first drug to combat high cholesterol was made and the first antibiotic to combat tuberculosis—had developed a drug to treat onchocerciasis, an awful disease that leads to irreversible blindness. At the time, CEO Dr. P. Roy Vagelos said the company would donate the drug, generically known as

Ivermectin, to countries that requested it. Donate, as in "give for free"! I was amazed and gratified.

River blindness, as the condition is commonly known, affects millions of people in West and Central Africa, the Middle East, and Central and South America. Caused by a parasitic worm, it is spread by the bite of certain blackflies. Although WHO had been working hard to eradicate the fly with insecticides, it was proving to be an expensive, impossible task in the long term, and the drug, although it couldn't cure the blind, changed the playing field for future generations. Senator Ted Kennedy of Massachusetts was so moved by the expensive gesture, he told a news conference: "Merck's gift to the World Health Organization is more than a medical breakthrough. It is truly a triumph of the human spirit."[39]

Kennedy's comment echoed my own sentiments back then. Now, fifteen years later, I was working on the global strategy for disease prevention and control, and was excited to come across such people again, impressive people who could bridge the public and private sectors in an effort to use their financial clout and intellectual heft to bring about change. No one personifies that commitment more for me than Lars Rebien Sørensen, then CEO of the Denmark-based multinational pharmaceutical company Novo Nordisk. He and his second-in-command, Dr. Stig Pramming, the company's senior medical director, became friends and heroes.

Sørensen told me about the moment he realized he was on the wrong side of the equation in the battle for public health.

During a visit to South Africa in the early 1990s, where he was representing the pharmaceutical industry as a whole, he was sitting across the table from President Mandela and listening to the litany of health challenges the country faced, including HIV/AIDS. He left impressed, and determined that Novo Nordisk, known for its manufacturing of insulin, needles, and all other things to treat diabetes, should become more socially responsible and work with the public sector in the drive to provide health services for all. Diabetes, he decided, would be the gateway through which his company would tackle all noncommunicable diseases. For him, as for Vagelos of Merck, the principal driving factors of a successful company were not—and should not be—profits and keeping shareholders happy. Sometimes, when you saw a need, you had to fill it. Be it drugs to help eradicate a parasitic illness that was destroying lives, reduced prices for insulin, or more funding devoted to increasing our knowledge of noncom-municable diseases—*our* knowledge, publicly accessible, not a company's tightly guarded secrets. When Novo Nordisk invested 40 per cent of the total cost in setting up a diabetes research center at Oxford University, its name was not on the center and it had no exclusive or patent rights to discoveries. Because that wasn't the point.

Because of that eureka moment with Mandela, Novo Nordisk funded the first conference in a series collectively called Oxford Vision 2020, which was dedicated to build-ing consensus and developing recommendations for a new and comprehensive approach to preventing and controlling chronic diseases, including diabetes. I sat on the board and was a member of the conference's planning committee.

Held at Magdalen College at Oxford University in December 2003, when I was still at WHO, it was chaired by John Bell, the Canadian-born immunologist and geneticist who had been appointed to Regius Professor of Medicine at Oxford the year before. One of the most remarkable things about the meeting was its diverse list of attendees. It drew from the worlds of public health, NGOs, and big business, from China to Scandinavia to the United States and the United Kingdom, all speaking to each other and forming relationships. Among them were Pramming and Niels Christiansen of Nestlé; Ruth Colagiuri of the Australian Centre for Diabetes Strategies; Dr. Chunming Chen, founding president of the Chinese Center for Disease Control and Prevention; and Dr. Philippe Halban, a medical professor at the University of Geneva and the director of Jeantet Research Laboratories.

Our goal was to place the prevention (and treatment) of noncommunicable diseases higher on the agendas of both governments and industries. At the Oxford Series conferences between 2004 and 2012, born of that first meeting in 2003, we accomplished much of what we set out to do. They helped to reinforce my belief that such partnerships can work, as long as both sides have similar goals and don't see each other as the enemy. The lessons I learned at that first conference helped me decide where I would land next.

■

As my work on the global strategy at WHO was winding down, I got a call from Dr. Michael Merson, then dean of public health at Yale University. He asked: "Would you be interested in coming to the university and joining our global health faculty, developing our first course in noncommunicable diseases in developing countries? It would be a tenured position."

I had no idea what a tenured position meant (something that would come back to haunt me). But Yale was where my long-time hero, Dr. Winslow, founded the public health program in the 1900s.

"That sounds nice," I said. "Let me talk it over with my wife."

It was a big decision. What would Yasmin do in the United States? What would the country be like? After Switzerland, after Geneva, where everything was so close, after Cape Town, with a community we both knew so well, America seemed distant and, well, foreign. We would have to make a new start, choose a town, buy a house, find a preschool for Julian, and build a whole new set of friends. There would be drivers' licenses to transfer (I would fail the first time), and I'd heard the traffic in major cities and on highways was so bad it was hard to gauge how long a trip would take.

In the end, though, we decided to go. To make a fresh start. Yale was Ivy League, the public health faculty was respected around the world, and I would be able to use my expertise to help make it a truly international program. And Yasmin, an epidemiologist who specialized in the environment and children's health, was able to transfer to the WHO office in New York.

For me, Yale would provide the opportunity to renew a friendship with Dr. Kelly Brownell, then chairman of the psychology department, who invented the terms "yo-yo dieting" and "toxic food environment." Gregarious, warm, and pudgy, he was beloved by his students, eloquent and concise when speaking to the media, and willing to discreetly give food companies advice on what they should be doing to avoid what was coming.

We had first met at WHO, when Bill Steiger of the US Department of Health and Human Services had written that thirty-page letter to Lee protesting the recommendations we made in the draft of our Global Strategy on Diet, Physical Activity, and Health. In response, Brownell and New York University nutrition professor Marion Nestle had agreed to co-write an op-ed in the *New York Times,* which ran on January 23, 2004. Obesity was a global epidemic, they warned, and governments—politicians—needed to stop the calculating trade of calories for dollars.

"That the food industry is disputing the WHO's science is all the more astonishing because the report is notable for the stunning banality of its dietary recommendations: eat more fruits and vegetables, and limit intake of foods high in fats and sugars," they wrote. "Such recommendations are no different from those issued by governments and health organizations since the late 1950's [*sic*] and are thoroughly supported by both science and common sense."[40]

Did it work? Maybe a bit. At least the strategy was approved by member states! And in Brownell, I found a kindred spirit, someone with whom I could eventually share everything—from concerns about the future to my frustration with a university bureaucracy that expected me to produce while setting roadblocks every step of the way. I had to wage fierce battles whenever I tried to enter the department into public-private partnerships, despite Yale having a long-established relationship with pharmaceutical company Pfizer Inc. What I wanted to do was different from what the school was accustomed to: I wanted to accept money from a pharmaceutical company not to do joint research but, rather, drive an "advocacy agenda" that was only indirectly related to its own interests.

In effect, I was trying to create a version of the Oxford Series at Yale, where people who tended to keep to their own circles would have the opportunity to talk to each other. The lesson I wanted to teach was one I already knew well: business can be an invaluable ally.

Brownell and I would work together in another key way, too, at Yale's Rudd Center for Food Policy and Obesity. Benefactor Leslie Rudd, a business magnate from Kansas who made his fortune in the food and beverage business, funded the nonprofit center as a hub through which we could work to study diet and activity patterns and hold industry and government agencies accountable for safeguarding and promoting public health. Overweight himself, Rudd, who counts the Dean & DeLuca upscale grocery stores among his holdings, wanted to reverse the global rates of obesity, reduce weight bias, and galvanize communities, public officials, and advocacy groups to achieve positive, lasting change. And he wanted my friend to head it.

Brownell brought me along as the head of the center's division for global health. It was a dream job, in that he always understood the importance of the public and private sectors working together to effect change. Although he was critical of business practices, he would never dismiss a business out of hand. Instead, he was always open to questions and giving advice; he wanted the division to act according to the strict standards he set himself.

Things were going well. However, even as I was becoming more skilled at negotiating academia, I realized that life with tenure was not for me. Before, I'd worked on teams to achieve my goals, from the National Health Centre in South Africa to the international tobacco control treaty and the global strategy for diet, physical activity, and health. I'd written scholarly papers with others and cooperated with experts around the world for the good of people in general. At Yale, as with many other universities, I was mostly on my own, rated on what *I* published, what speeches *I* gave, and any other accomplishments *I* made—and even though I could more than hold my own in that department, it wasn't what I was interested in doing. Sometimes, it was a bit like swimming with sharks, an activity I had already done in real life back in South Africa. There was a trick to it. You had to swim steadily, eyes straight ahead, but always, always aware of exactly what was going on around you. And then in 2005, Michael Merson, who'd invited me to come Yale in the first place, lost a battle to separate the School of Public Health from the School of Medicine and announced he was leaving for Duke University in Durham, North Carolina, to become the founding director of the Duke Global Health Institute.

It was a rocky time in the department, with lots of loud consternation and behind-the-scenes muttering about what the future held there—and I soon realized it was time for me to go. To put it bluntly, I wasn't happy.

The timing couldn't have been better. Toward the end of the 2004–05 academic year, I got a call from Judith Rodin, the new president of the Rockefeller Foundation.

"Would you like to join us as our global health director?" she asked.

At first glance, the Rockefeller Foundation seemed right up my alley. The private foundation was begun in 1913 by John D. Rockefeller Sr., who owned Standard Oil; his son, John D. Rockefeller Jr.; and Frederick Taylor Gates, a Baptist clergyman and Sr.'s principal business and philanthropic advisor. According to its charter, its mission is to promote "the well-being of humanity throughout the world." The organization represented the epitome of efforts being made in global health, a level that others could only try to aspire to, a driving force in the field for nearly a century. It helped to establish the London School of Hygiene & Tropical Medicine in the United Kingdom, the School of Hygiene at the University of Toronto, the Harvard School of Public Health, and my own alma mater at Johns Hopkins. Numerous other accomplishments included developing a vaccine against yellow fever and helping to provide a haven at The New School in New York City for scholars who'd been forced flee Nazi Germany.

In the 1960s and '70s, it was the largest funder of groundbreaking health initiatives outside government-run organizations; others didn't even come close. And in 2005, when Rodin called me, the foundation had donated $3 million to build housing for victims of Hurricane Katrina in New Orleans and another $8 million to develop microbicides to help stem the transmission of the HIV virus and ensure their easy availability to women in developing countries.

I'd been involved with the foundation before, too. As the representative from South Africa, I'd been included in a high-level meeting about the future of WHO in 1995, just before Yasmin and I left Cape Town for Geneva. The meeting was held at Kykuit, the neoclassical estate (and national landmark) that John D. Rockefeller built in Sleepy Hollow, New York. I'd also attended a number of think tanks at the foundation-owned Bellagio Center, a fifty-acre estate on the shore of Lake Como in northern Italy, including one in June 1995 on the implications of global trends in tobacco control and consumption. Although the meeting took place before we began to work on the global tobacco control treaty, most of the same people involved in it were there. As the foundation approached its centenary, I saw the job offer as a once-in-a-lifetime chance to join the celebration and contribute to what it would become over the next hundred years.

I told Rodin I would be delighted to join the foundation.

I think I gave Yale only two weeks' notice.

■

From my twenty-eighth-storey office in the foundation's gorgeous high-rise building on Fifth Avenue, I looked down and saw a line of yellow taxis stretching into the distance, jostling umbrellas, and endless streams of people. New York was a city on the move and so was I.

Or so I thought.

About a year after I joined, Warren Buffett, the billionaire investor and philanthropist, pledged $31 billion to the Bill & Melinda Gates Foundation, making it the richest and most powerful foundation in the world. There was a lively ceremony at the New York Public Library, where Buffett signed the papers handing over his shares in his Berkshire Hathaway holding company to that foundation (and an additional $6 billion to four others).

"How wonderful that two of the planet's richest men are coming together in the name of global health," I was moved to tell staff afterwards.

They all looked at me in horror. "But where does it leave us?" I was asked. "We're no longer a serious player!"

All of a sudden, I understood that many of them had become so consumed with funding and with the visibility given the foundation's projects in the media that they had lost sight of its larger mission. It didn't matter when the Gates Foundation, which had been started in 2000, reached out to our own and said we were still the major player in global health, with the most experience and deepest understanding. The decision was made: we could no longer compete in that field because we didn't have that kind of money. We'd have to find something else—causes such as "resilience-building," in which communities and countries are given the means to withstand environmental disasters such as earthquakes. With my public health expertise and emphasis on prevention, I didn't fit in.

Instead of helping shape the foundation's legacy for the next one hundred years, I found myself stymied at every turn. Suggestions were rejected. Money was scarce. It all came to a head in the summer of 2006, when I tried to organize a meeting at the Bellagio Center for the heads of a number of foundations about how to best address the issue of non-communicable diseases at the international level. Working together, I thought we'd be stronger. With that in mind, on July 26, I wrote an e-mail to Robert Beaglehole, a New Zealand public health expert who at the time was the director of one of the noncommunicable disease groups at WHO.

"Internally, the going is tough," I said. "You could help by having Kenya and Thai colleagues start pressuring the RF regional offices in Nairobi and Bangkok."

Two days later—a Friday—the foundation's general counsel called me to come into the office immediately. When I got there, Rodin was on the phone from the Bellagio Center.

They told me I was dismissed for insubordination, that I was trying to influence the board and the foundation to go in a direction that ran counter to what I believed should be its very mission: to help the poorest of the poor.

It was one of the worst moments in my career. I couldn't believe what I was hearing, not because I had an overweening ego but because I was being fired for doing what I had always done. Noncommunicable diseases were my specialty. Tobacco, obesity, and everything that stemmed from them—lung cancer, heart disease, and type 2 diabetes among them—might not discriminate between social strata, but they are killers nonetheless. Of the rich and the poor. Of people in developed and developing countries. For *this,* I was losing my job?

"You'll be formally dismissed on Monday," I was told.

I walked out of the office, seething.

Call a labor lawyer, I told myself. Find out what your rights are.

The first thing the labor lawyer told me was that the foundation was perfectly within its legal rights to fire me since I was not a member of a union and didn't have protective clauses in my contract. But—and this was a big but—it was taking a morally and ethically ridiculous position, never mind an overreaction of gigantic proportions. We formed a plan, which I honed over the weekend.

Remain calm, I kept repeating to myself. Matter-of-factly state your case and act like you won't take no for an answer.

When I went to see the foundation counsel that Monday morning, I said that if they went through with my firing, the repercussions would be profound. "Profound" is such a good word, at once scary and open-ended. I said that my very life in the United States was at stake because I was on a visa that required I work in academia or for a nonprofit organization. If I lost my job, the foundation would have to deal with the fallout of dismissing an international expert, one of the architects of both the Framework Convention on Tobacco Control and the Global Strategy on Diet, Physical Activity and Health. I had managed to place these issues on the agenda of the World Health Organization, yet was being prevented from continuing that important work here.

This wasn't a time for acronyms. Everything was spelled out to emphasize the import of my message.

The answer came immediately.

"Okay," I was told. "We'll give you an extension for however long it takes you to find something else."

In the interim, Rodin allowed me to be seconded full-time to the Clinton Global Initiative, which I continued to work with until it was shut down during the 2016 US election campaign. At the time, one of its areas of focus was global health, not in a big-picture, hazy kind of way but rather working to persuade governments and private industry to come together to tackle major social issues in specific communities and countries. Merck, for example—the same company that developed the drug to combat river blindness and distributed it for free to any country that asked for it—provided enough of the Gardasil vaccine against the human papillomavirus, which can cause cervical cancer, to protect all the girls in Colombia. The effort was not without controversy. Some people, many of them opposed to vaccinations in general, claimed the vaccine caused some girls to faint or become ill, and in August 2017, a class action lawsuit was filed against the Colombian government and the pharmaceutical company.

My job was to help insure that there was real substance and intent to each company's proposal. After the Rockefeller Foundation, it was a wonderful experience to have prevention and public health all rolled up into one good cause. I was happy there, but I knew I had to move on, as I was still ostensibly a Rockefeller Foundation employee. It wanted me gone and I needed to go.

A couple of months after I started at the initiative, my cell phone rang. It was the office of Indra Nooyi, PepsiCo's incoming CEO. Would it be possible for me to join her for lunch later that week?

"Sure," I said. Calls like this were not out of the norm. Sometimes, food company executives had questions or needed clarifications. I thought Nooyi probably wanted to have an informal chat about nutrition. She, however, had something else in mind.

7

OPENING UP A CAN OF TROUBLE

One week after Nooyi's phone call, I headed from our home in Southport, Connecticut, to PepsiCo's world headquarters in Purchase, New York. It was going to be a very busy few days.

I had a lunch with Nooyi at noon and would be catching a flight from LaGuardia to Minneapolis for a meeting the next morning—and probably a job offer from Lois Quam, CEO of Ovations, an innovative branch of the UnitedHealth Group. The company had earmarked $15 million for developing countries so they could better deal with cardiovascular and sexually transmitted diseases.

Sandwiched between Pepsi and LaGuardia, at 2:30 p.m., I'd participate in a panel discussion on Minnesota Public Radio about diet, health, and the perils of big food companies. I'd been invited to take part after the journal *Nature* published a paper I'd written with Kelly Brownell and Dr. David Stuckler titled "Epidemiological and Economic Consequences of the Global Epidemics of Obesity and Diabetes." The other guest was Michele Simon, a public health lawyer who specialized in legal strategies to counter corporate tactics and who had just published a book called *Appetite for Profit: How the Food Industry Undermines Our Health and How to Fight Back.*

Oh God. I'll have to ask if I can borrow an office to do the public radio panel, I thought, as I drove to meet Nooyi. *How weird is that—discussing the dangers of big food companies from Pepsi headquarters?*

I'd given myself lots of time for the drive. If there was one thing I'd learned since coming to the United States, it was the perils of gridlock, no matter how near or far your destination. Although Purchase, in leafy Westchester County, was only twenty-seven miles from our house on Wakeman Lane, if there was an accident, or semi-trailers using the passing lane, or just one very slow driver, the journey could take an hour and a half, maybe longer. There was no way I was going to be late!

Along the way, I had time to think about the first (and only) time I'd met Nooyi. There was a "top-to-top" meeting in Prague eighteen months earlier, just as I was leaving Yale for the Rockefeller Foundation. Brock Leach, a PepsiCo executive I'd met during the talks with multinational food companies during the drawing up of the WHO guidelines on nutrition and health, called to invite me to a very high-level private confab convened by his boss, PepsiCo CEO Steve Reinemund. He wanted me to speak about my experience at WHO and to offer my opinion on what the food industry might do.

Henry Kissinger was there, as was former Israeli prime minister Ehud Barak and Dr. Dean Ornish, the doctor who put former US president Bill Clinton on his diet and was already the chair of a PepsiCo Blue Ribbon Advisory Board tasked with advising the company on how to make its products healthier. Nooyi attended and I went with Yasmin.

Our encounter was brief and breezy, handshakes all around accompanied by general talk about food, WHO, and promises to meet again in the future. Back then, she was in charge of the company's corporate strategy, a tall, elegant, independent woman who was preparing for the future, not three or five years down the road but in the much longer term. Her job was to figure out what PepsiCo would look like in twenty or thirty years, and to make both employees and consumers believe in her vision.

Now, she was poised to step into the top job, and I was curious. What was her vision?

That will be my first question.

■

I was escorted to Nooyi's office, where a wall of glass that looked out over a man-made lake, rolling green fields, and the Donald M. Kendall Sculpture Gardens, a collection of forty-five outdoor sculptures by Auguste Rodin, Henry Moore, and Joan Miró, among others. They seemed the backdrop to our meeting inside: silent, angular, and immutable. At first, I couldn't take my eyes off them.

Nooyi invited me to sit at a table where we could talk—chitchat at first as we got comfortable with each other. I told her a story about the night we met, when Yasmin and I were seated at a table with her husband and Kissinger. My father-in-law, Kurt von Schirnding, a diplomat and South African ambassador to the United Nations in the 1980s, had frequently disagreed with the policies of Prime Minister P.W. Botha. He was celebrating his seventy-fifth birthday that day, and I asked Kissinger, whom he idolized, to write him a note.

"It was the best present my father-in-law ever got, I think," I said.

We spoke about Yale and my friend Kelly Brownell, whom Nooyi thought had "great integrity." After about fifteen minutes, an aide brought in a cart set with plates of grilled salmon and assorted vegetables, a basket of bread rolls, and a selection of drinks from PepsiCo's portfolio. Given where I was, I briefly considered choosing a Pepsi but opted for iced tea.

As we began to eat, we finally got down to the conversation that had been hovering at the edges, waiting like a thief to break in.

"Tell me," I said, "what is your vision for the company?"

Nooyi took her time in answering. What finally came out was a story of growing up in a Brahmin family in Chennai, or Madras as it was then known, on the Bay of Bengal. Of going to the best schools in India, of seeing lineups that, to her young eyes, did not end. Of people waiting for rice for their families and crying because they were hungry. As a child, she dreamed of making it better. Now, as the incoming CEO of PepsiCo, she had the tools to try.

"I want to tackle undernutrition," she said. "What would it take for people at WHO to take us more seriously?"

"I'm not sure," I replied, my mind racing. I wasn't prepared for a question quite like this! "Engaging with NGOs or UN agencies is, admittedly, a challenge for you. You're seen as bad people who are trying to stop us from doing our job. You're seen as not taking obesity seriously."

"But I do. *We* do" came her answer. "You asked what my vision is. My vision is to transform this company into a healthier company—and I want you to help me do it."

I nearly choked on a mouthful of salmon and could feel my face flushing red as a beetroot, my body's automatic response to being caught completely off guard. Nooyi had definitely done just that.

"Well, what do you think?" she prompted.

"I … I don't know what to say," I sputtered. "Honestly, I came here because I thought you just wanted a general chat about nutrition."

She didn't miss a beat. "As you can see, that's not the case. I want you to do exactly what you were doing at WHO before you left and do it here for us at PepsiCo," she said.

"Derek, I'm asking you to come join us. Fight the fight from the inside."

I sat back in my chair, feeling clammy. *Was that my heart going* ka-THUNK? "I ... uh ... I need a bit of time to think about it," I replied. "Is it okay if I get back to you at the beginning of next week?"

"Of course!" she said.

Knowing about the interview I was to do on the Minnesota Public Radio broadcast, she then had staff take me to an office, where I sat perfectly still for about twenty minutes, trying to compose myself. When the station called my cell in advance of the panel discussion, the mischievous little boy in me was tempted to blurt out, "Guess where I am!" But I didn't. There would be plenty of criticism levied against me if I accepted Nooyi's offer, so why start then? I made it through the twenty-minute discussion unscathed, answering questions about popular diets and making my opinions known in a manner that somehow sounded reasonable and intelligent.

Afterwards, I retrieved my coat and walked out of the building, cautious, excited, and terrified all at once. On the one hand, there was no job description. I would have free rein to create and tailor it as I saw fit, a health advisor who would have the power of the CEO of a major multinational company behind me. Nooyi insisted she didn't want me to edit myself. She wanted to know what I really thought and wanted me to think outside the box.

On the other hand, I could imagine what colleagues would say.

Sell-out.

Defector.

Turncoat.

How could *you?*

As soon as I'd pulled out of the PepsiCo parking lot, I called Yasmin from the car to tell her what had happened. "Are you crazy?" she said. "Derek, that is not a good idea."

Yet I couldn't stop thinking about it on the drive to LaGuardia Airport.

At PepsiCo, you won't have to build a consensus between competing factions. It's not WHO, with member states with different interests. Or at least it won't be up to you to build that consensus.

And: *Would I have a chance to be more effective by being an inside man?*

I wasn't being naive. I knew there would be marketing and sales departments to placate and bring over to my side, but they weren't like governments, countries, with a host of other interests, including elections, to consider. For the first time since Gro Harlem Brundtland brought me on to her WHO management team and appointed me director of the Tobacco Free Initiative, it felt like there was someone who would have my back, no matter what others thought of my position. And I wouldn't be starting from zero: the company already had its Blue Ribbon Advisory Panel that included Ornish and Brundtland, which had recommended that PepsiCo eliminate all trans fats from its products. Starting in 2003, it became the first mainstream company to begin to do so.

I could deal with that, couldn't I?

When I got to my hotel room in Minnetonka, twenty miles southwest of Minneapolis, I called Yasmin again. The more we talked about it that night and again the next morning, the more compelling the offer became. Could I really refuse to work for a company that wanted to transform itself and wanted to hire me to achieve that goal? Was it that unthinkable a notion? Or—better question—was it more unthinkable to not even try?

At the same time, I tried to prepare for the meeting with Lois Quam at Ovations. I suspected I knew what she wanted to talk about. Three years earlier, when I was at Yale, I'd helped her put together the $15-million package for developing countries, and we'd coauthored a piece, "Rising to the Global Challenge of Chronic Diseases," that would be published in *The Lancet* that year (2006). Now, it was time to build the program to scale and create a network to support it, and she wanted me to run it.

In the space of less than a week, I went from no jobs on the horizon to considering two. One involved trying to change the culture from the inside of one of the biggest companies in the world; the other meant continuing what I had begun as an epidemiologist back in South Africa, only on a much larger scale.

All I knew of Minnesota was what I'd heard from Garrison Keillor and *A Prairie Home Companion*, his sly, folksy weekly program on NPR. Was there really a Lake Wobegon, where he professed to live? I didn't think so, but I suspected there were lots of place like that here—places where the wind howled in off the lakes in winter, the summers were humid and buggy, and neighbors were mostly willing to lend a hand. Could I be happy here? More important, could Yasmin and our son be happy here?

I don't think so.

At the time I'd accepted Quam's invitation to meet, there'd been nothing else on the immediate horizon, and the Rockefeller Foundation wanted me to find something fast. As much as I liked and respected her, and as interesting as the job might be, it was really a continuation of the work I'd been doing for much of my life, most recently at Yale.

PepsiCo seemed so much bigger, so much more challenging.

After the meeting, I turned right around, flew back to New York, picked up the car at the airport garage, and made a beeline for home. I was going to work at the second-biggest multinational food and beverage company in the world!

■

"Are you sure?" Nooyi asked.

"I think so," I said.

Before I formally accepted the as-yet-to-be-defined position, she wanted me to realize in no uncertain terms what I would be up against: she arranged for me to meet with Reinemund, the outgoing CEO who'd organized that meeting in Prague. I sat down in his office, and without any ceremony, he plunked a bag of Doritos on the big desk between us.

"Before you join the company, how are you going to defend the fact that we make this?" he asked. "How are you going to defend that your salary is partly based on the fact that the company makes this stuff until such time as we produce only healthy products?"

The brutally frank questions stopped me cold. I'd be working for the company that made Pepsi, Cheetos, Tostitos, Doritos, and Cap'n Crunch cereal, among other high-fat, high-sodium, high-sugar products. My paycheque would say "PepsiCo" on it. Could I accept that and still do the best job I could? A phrase we used in South Africa came to mind: *They had to rewire the plane after apartheid and keep the plane flying while they were doing it.* PepsiCo had to do the same thing: rewire itself while depending on a profit stream that depended on foods and drinks that weren't healthy.

Working there would be a delicate balancing act on a number of fronts, within the company and without—and within my own battling conscience. I knew I was tough. I had always gone my own way when I was convinced I was right, no matter the pressure or the price that I paid. Back in 2004, I'd left WHO because of a sustained, expensive effort by the sugar industry to get rid of me after I had the temerity to suggest that consumers limit their sugar intake. If there was one thing I'd learned from that experience, it was that public health and nutrition professionals had to enter a sustained dialogue with the food industry to effect change. And now, I was being given an incredible opportunity to work from the inside, provided I had the backbone to withstand the inevitable criticism from my peers.

So far, my career had been a rocky one because of the goals I was always trying to achieve, which were unpopular in some powerful quarters. It had been marked by winning, then losing, and winning and losing again—and I'd survived. At that moment, I was most unhappy at the Rockefeller Foundation (and they were less and less happy at me being there). I felt the foundation had lost its way in its impossible scramble to keep up with the Gates Foundation Joneses and was blocking me from doing my job. Never mind that in South Africa under apartheid rule, I'd developed a very thick skin, its color alone having led to my being ostracized by the rest of the world for a good chunk of my career.

I could hear my father whispering to me: *You grew up swimming your own race at your own pace, against tides and whitecap waves. Why stop yourself now?*

"That's a good question," I finally told Reinemund. "But I've learned through my career to be patient and focus on what's important, no matter the outside pressures. I know there will be pressure here, and lots of shock and vehement disapproval from elsewhere. I can handle it." Even as I said it, I started to believe it. I knew that this job, more than any other thus far, would be so challenging, different, and potentially life changing, that it was impossible to resist.

I framed it to others, to my mother, my siblings, and friends, in more pragmatic terms. I chose to try to make a difference for the billions of people who consumed PepsiCo products year after year after year.

I called Quam to let her know something else had come up. "Oh?" she said. "What?"

When I told her, she was surprised but understood why. I wasn't saying no to joining her but, rather, saying yes to something completely different.

"Good luck—and just make sure you go in with your eyes open," she said.

"Don't worry," I said. "I will."

■

Once the news broke, the disapprobation came quickly. Dr. Marion Nestle, NYU professor, author of *Food Politics*, and nutrition blogger, to whom I had turned for support during the fight over the global diet strategy at WHO, told an interviewer from NPR: "I couldn't believe it. I was really astounded. I mean, it's not like he went to work for a company that's selling carrots. He went to work for a company that's selling sugar water!"[41] She believed the best thing PepsiCo could do for the food industry was to go out of business altogether.

Nestle's sentiments were echoed by people such as Michele Simon, with whom I'd appeared on the Minnesota Public Radio show while at PepsiCo headquarters, and by lots—and *lots*—of former colleagues, including Dr. Kaare R. Norum, professor emeritus in the Department of Nutrition at the University of Oslo. I'd been co-opted, they said. It was a public relations coup for PepsiCo and a black mark on my reputation as an expert who had previously pressured food companies to stop marketing junk food to kids.

Had I been hired for the optics? That may have been part of Nooyi's motivation, but it certainly wasn't that alone. Long before I first met her in Prague, she had organized the sale in 1997 of PepsiCo's fast-food divisions such as Pizza Hut, Taco Bell, and KFC, and, three years later, had overseen the purchase of companies with more health-friendly product lines, including Quaker Oats and Tropicana. There was already intent and a track record. I was brought on to make sense of the enormous ferment going on inside the company, which was unseen by outside observers, and to map growth opportunities for the future.

■

The first challenge was getting a new visa to live and work in the United States. Until then, I'd been in the United States on an H-1B visa as a specialty worker for a nonprofit company. Yale qualified, as did the Rockefeller Foundation. Obviously,

PepsiCo did not. Now, I had to apply for an 0-1 visa, granted to aliens with "extraordinary ability" in the arts, education, business, athletics, or, in my case, sciences. In the petition, the company had to show that, as a pioneer in the field of global health policy, I would bring an exceptional talent to the United States that would undoubtedly benefit American citizens. The petition had to contain five letters of support from influential, independent experts in a position to evaluate what I had done to merit such a job offer. But by joining PepsiCo, I, the alien applicant for an 0-1 visa, had effectively alienated many colleagues in the communities of public health and nutrition. Who could I turn to for support?

I reached out to people like Dr. Pekka Puska, who'd worked with me on WHO's draft guidelines for food and nutrition and was now director-general of the National Public Health Institute of Finland; Dr. Julio Frenk, a former minister of health in Mexico; and Dr. Ricardo Uauy, president of the International Union of Nutritional Sciences and a professor in both the Institute of Nutrition and Food Technology at the University of Chile and the London School of Hygiene & Tropical Medicine.

In his letter, Uauy wrote: "I rank Derek Yach in the top 5 per cent of the academics I have met in the field, especially considering his impact on policy implementation based on the best available science. His extraordinary expertise and leadership skills are well-known and often sought out throughout the world by international and Bilateral Agencies in the area of food and nutrition."[42]

Following his letter of recommendation, Uauy insisted on coming to Nooyi's office to meet with both of us. Burly, with white thinning hair, a trim beard, and thick eyebrows that spoke a language all their own, he sat down, reached into his jacket pocket, and pulled out a handful of seeds that turned out to be quinoa.

"Here's the problem," he said. "I just got back from Bolivia and the people there want to trade their seeds for Pepsi and Coke. How do you stop them from trading a nutritious crop for bad stuff?"

"PepsiCo simply has to make nutritious foods as attractive as everything else," Nooyi replied.

Training his eyes—and those eyebrows—on her, he continued: "Derek is our standard-bearer in the fight against chronic diseases, so I hope you're not going to turn him into a shill, defending the indefensible."

Nooyi laughed. "Listen, Ricardo, the minute he goes native, he's out of here. He is of value to us only so long as he continues to call things as he sees them and to remind us that we need to change. His job is to steer that change."

Neither one asked what I thought. It was strange to have these two forceful, charismatic characters speak about me and my future as if I wasn't there.

After that meeting, Uauy wrote an editorial in the scientific journal *Public Health Nutrition* saying that he believed in me and what I wanted to do.[43] In the same issue, Norum, of the University of Oslo, provided a counterpoint, writing that the very premise of changing industry from the inside was flawed. "Branding snacks as healthy only diverts attention from the real issues ... In my view, it is the culture of snacking—the consumption of superfluous calories between, or perhaps instead of healthy main meals—which is an unhealthy practice in itself."[44]

The journal gave me space in the same issue to respond to Norum and Uauy and defend my decision. I wrote that my experience at WHO had convinced me that there had to be a dialogue with the food companies. Their industry, with all its facets and products, wasn't at all like tobacco, which marketed a single carcinogenic product that we could easily classify as dangerous. As I had stressed during my initial dinner with Nestlé's Niels Christiansen on that autumn evening back in 2002, food companies were different because they offered myriad products, some of which were more dangerous to people's health than others. There were sodium levels to consider, and sugar and fat.[45]

But if Nooyi was to be believed, it was a dizzying, exciting challenge. How could I have said no?

8

INSIDE MAN
AT PEPSI

Never censor myself. For the nearly five years I worked at PepsiCo, that was my mantra. Most of the time, I was comfortable, even serene, in the knowledge that I was working to change a food company while at same time accepting a pay cheque from it. I began to build the parameters of a job where the description, if there had been one, would have read: Change a behemoth, one excruciatingly small step at a time.

I took Nooyi at her word and always made sure to put forth the strongest case for self-transformation and the negative effects of current products. I gave presentations about the burden of disease and death caused by obesity. In the meetings, PepsiCo marketers did not take kindly to the mentions of disease, death, and Doritos in the same sentence. They

133

134 DR. DEREK YACH

balked at my suggestion that the products were unhealthy and a cause of obesity, with all that condition's accompanying health problems. They didn't want to know about type 2 diabetes or heart disease. Instead, they suggested people needed to get out more, walk along a beach, cycle with their kids, play a game of pickup basketball or shinny. It wasn't "us." It was "them." Consumers bore responsibility for their health and well-being, and PepsiCo simply made products that they happened to find delicious.

Freedom of choice, right? But I'd heard that argument before.

There was a stigma against the obese, I argued. They were judged on sight, convicted of being lazy, and sentenced to endure the thinner public's contempt, yet tackling the problem and achieving optimum health for all should be a co-operative effort. We had a responsibility to help. We had to change the fact that junk food was much cheaper to buy than fresh food; develop new, lower-priced products to fill a void; and work with the public to improve their lifestyles. We had to set the example. As I had learned at WHO, the food industry wasn't in the same league as tobacco at all. Tobacco was easy to categorize as dangerous. Food was not. There would always be naysayers. At times, I had to ask myself if it was all worth it— especially when I found myself experiencing the second academic boycott of my career. When I worked in South Africa, most journal editors outside the country's borders refused to publish my work because of the color of my skin. Now, no matter how rigorous the methodology of my papers, many journals shunned me because I had gone to work for a company that made products considered detrimental to the public's health. Two examples stand out in my mind.

Initially, *BMJ*, formerly the *British Medical Journal*, invited me to write a major review about the potential for private food companies to address undernutrition around the world. When I submitted it, the editor wrote back to say that it sounded too positive about the private sector and wouldn't be going out for peer review. Well, obviously, I was going to write a positive article! I'd gone to work for PepsiCo, for goodness sakes. Eventually, the article was published in the *American Journal of Public Health*, which has one of the toughest article standards in the world.

The second example was even more bizarre. Knowing full well where I worked, editors at the *Journal of the American Medical Association* (*JAMA*) asked me to write a piece about obesity, in collaboration with Marion Nestle of NYU and David Ludwig, a professor of nutrition at Harvard University. The three of us agreed and began to lay out ideas on how (or if) the public and private sectors could ever find common ground. I had no expectations that Nestle would understand my point of view, but I was glad that I was being given the opportunity to argue my case in a professional journal. In the end, though, *JAMA* actually turned down my article because it apparently reflected the private sector in too positive a light, and Nestle and Ludwig ended up doing the project on their own. Certainly, it was disappointing, but I couldn't lose sight of why I had come to PepsiCo in the first place: Nooyi's powerful message that corporations could, and should, instigate and enforce positive change.

In 2006, under Nooyi, PepsiCo had rebranded itself as "Performance with Purpose"—a company with a conscience that was focused on delivering sustainable long-term growth and leaving a positive imprint on society and the environment. Michael Porter, a Harvard economist, had outlined the principles of that idea in a speech at the Prague meeting where I'd first met Nooyi; in 2011, they would be enshrined in the *Harvard Business Review* in an article titled "Creating Shared Value."

That's what Nooyi was determined to do. In the '90s, 100 per cent of PepsiCo's US portfolio was labeled "Fun for You" treats. By 2008, Nooyi was able to tell a Food Marketing Institute conference that the transformation of PepsiCo's product portfolio was well underway.

"We've accomplished this transformation by reformulating our existing products to make them healthier—for example, by eliminating trans fats altogether and switching to healthier ingredients like heart-healthy oils," she said at the conference. "We've also focused on growing new products with a healthier profile, such as baked snacks and diet drinks; and launched new products like Flat Earth, which contain a half serving of fruits or vegetables in every ounce of crisps, or G2, a half-calorie Gatorade. So, you see, it can be done."[46]

In her previous job as the chief of corporate strategy, Nooyi had articulated her global vision with clear long-term goals and had started to do that as best she could with the sell-off of businesses such as KFC and the purchase of others regarded as healthier. Now, the first challenge was to see if there were growth opportunities for the future.

That focus made my job different from that of the Blue Ribbon Advisory Panel. We set up new advisory boards made up of some of our toughest critics, asking them to speak to Nooyi and the PepsiCo board about what we needed to do to change. Basically, their message was that we needed to focus on consumers' health and well-being—a very different message for marketing and sales people accustomed to promoting good taste and enjoyment. I turned to a remarkable woman for help: Erika Karp. At that time, she was managing director of UBS, a global financial services company; she would go on to found Cornerstone Capital Group. She taught me to use the terms "corporate sustainability" and "corporate excellence" interchangeably. And she reinforced my belief that promoting the health and well-being of consumers and treating the environment with respect were as important as the almighty financial bottom line and would only help us in the long run. Karp posed the question: How do we place our investments to ensure not only their long-term survival and growth but also that of people? Although capitalism was still the best system, it was more effective when used to accomplish multipronged goals that might not seem related at first.

Sustainable agriculture and tackling obesity counted as much as—if not, in the long run, more than—buying, selling, or holding a company stock. In a keynote address to the tenth annual Business & Society Conference, Tuck School of Business at Darmouth in Hanover, New Hampshire, I described the progress we were making on several fronts.

"Increasingly our teams understand how shifts in the nutrient profile of foods and beverages create new business opportunities," I said. "We were well placed to take advantage of our food formulation work over years in Mexico when a new law requiring stricter standards on school meals came into force. And many of our advances in reducing fossil fuel use in our large truck fleet; in approaching zero waste; avoiding national electrical grid use; and attaining positive water balance in our Frito Lay California plant are actively sought after by other companies."[47]

Given the conference theme, "Trading Off: Impactful Business Strategies in Uncertain Times," I wanted to press home the point that corporate sustainability may be complicated, but if you're really committed and not just giving it short shrift for appearance's sake, it can actually spur profits, not deter them.

Of course, outside PepsiCo, it was frustrating to keep running up against academics who saw our world in black and white—much as I perceived tobacco companies. Sugar was bad, green leafy vegetables were good. And any product made by a company that was known for its soda and chips had to be bad, too. When PepsiCo's Tropicana division came up with a fruit puree for kids that was 99 per cent free of added sugar, NYU's Marion Nestle responded in hostile fashion on her blog, claiming we were "snackifying" and "drinkifying" a commercial product, which would be detrimental to their ability to enjoy fruit in the long term. The product, she concluded, had no redeemable quality.[48] I'll never forget what happened after. When I called her, she admitted she had never seen the product, never mind tasted it. The blog entry was just her take on what had already been written by others! I was quite shocked by that. However, she did agree to come speak to the head of Tropicana, who was distraught by her criticism because he was committed to making healthy products for children. Although she claimed to us that she came out of the meeting with a deeper understanding of what it takes to make products healthier, she bluntly said she would not write a retraction because that wasn't her job.

Undaunted and determined, we continued to come up with new product lines, among them the Sabra line of Middle Eastern dips, yogurt, and lower-fat and -sodium potato chips. To promote a healthier lifestyle, we reduced portion sizes and calorie counts. And we decided to form a separate branch of the company to address nutrition and health: we called it Nutrico. As a sign of the changing times, we were flooded with requests from younger employees who wanted to come work for it.

But the question Nooyi had posed during the lunch when she asked me to join the company kept coming back to haunt me: *What would it take to get WHO to take us seriously?* The answer to that question remained elusive. I realized that one company, or even two or three companies, would be hard pressed to do it on their own, because no matter their good intentions, they would be destroyed competitively in the market, outpriced and outmaneuvered. But if a group of multinational food companies joined together and showed a common front, we could both effect change more efficiently and engage WHO in our mission.

We figured we needed at least eight multinational companies to get involved and support the transformative issues we put on the table. Few had the vision of Nooyi and PepsiCo, although Unilever came close. Coca-Cola didn't want to rock the boat, while Kraft had a history of being owned by tobacco companies that had bucked any kind of change for years.

In the end, nine multinationals agreed to join us and create the International Food and Beverage Alliance—an NGO that would allow us to have a strong common voice and to work together in a noncompetitive way, starting with reducing the marketing of products to kids. The alliance tried to involve WHO, because we needed the organization to assess if what we were doing was working. But the comments that kept coming back to the alliance—such as "Reduce your marketing to kids," which we were already doing—indicated that WHO hadn't read the alliance's mandate or the documents sent. I don't know if it was due to lack of staff or simply lack of interest.

Meanwhile, in 2011, in conjunction with the World Food Programme and the US Agency for International Development, we began one of the most exciting pilot projects I have ever been involved with—one that I hoped would go a long way toward improving nutrition and health in Africa. It started when the government in Ethiopia wondered why the World Food Programme was bringing in Plumpy'Nut, a peanut-based product, when about 100,000 Ethiopian farmers grew chickpeas as a secondary crop. Could chickpeas be turned into a similar product? Our role was twofold: to develop a chickpea-based nutritional supplement and to work with Ethiopian farmers to increase production and quality, in effect making chickpeas their primary crop.

To me, the project was a perfect example of private and public interests working together to create a sustainable source of food in a country that has known drought and famine and would probably know them again. The nexus between profitability and development encapsulated what I was referring to in my keynote speech at Tuck School of Business at Dartmouth: "Increasingly our teams understand how shifts in the nutrient profile of foods and beverages create new business opportunities."[49]

Change would come and so would profit. But it would take time. We needed to give the program time to develop properly so that the seemingly disparate end goals—a populace with healthy food it could afford and benefits to company shareholders—could come together.

■

It would not turn out the way I hoped. Two years after the project started, company officials began asking me questions about it.

"Why did you use this NGO?"

"Why did you buy these chickpeas?"

I answered the questions as best I could, all the while mystified as to why they were being asked at all. Did someone complain? It was as if my responses were traveling down a black hole. Then, as abruptly as it started, it ended. Although it wasn't a formal investigation, the experience left me feeling disappointed, even bereft. A project that had been started with such hopes would now continue in a different iteration without me. As would PepsiCo. I knew that my career at the company had come to an end. I had done all I could. The inquiry had made me stressed and anxious. I found myself looking at colleagues and wondering: "Was it you who raised concerns?" It was a constant and daily refrain running in my head.

One morning at 6:30, Nooyi summoned me to her office. I was in early after a swim, as was my habit. At the time, she was in the midst of a shareholder revolt that was calling into question her direction and leadership and would last, off and on, for over two years. In the end, she would prevail, but there were times when she needed reassurance that she was doing the right thing—like on that day.

I told her she was, and not to stop. I also told her that the time had come for me to leave. I agreed to stay until the immediate shareholder crisis was resolved, which took several more months. Then I sat down to write a good-bye letter to the staff.

I said it had been a privilege to be part of the early development of the global R & D team, to help shape a set of nutrition goals that would guide future product decisions, to work with teams bridging the agriculture-nutrition and food divide, and to have the freedom to build new models for private-public collaboration. Despite my views often challenging their status quo, they readily accepted that there was a difference between intent to change and making it happen, not just once but on a sustained basis. We tried, and sometimes we succeeded.

"It is now time for me to move toward a new relationship with PepsiCo," I concluded. "It will be an ongoing privilege to serve the company in an advisory role while I start work on a new and exciting venture."

I was about to help people change their lives for the better from yet another vantage point, not quite outside and not quite in. I would become the quintessential middleman.

9

THE VIRTUOUS CYCLE

In South Africa and at WHO, my work was steeped in the public sector and its power to set the tone in prevention and health promotion among whole populations. At PepsiCo, I tackled a rising obesity epidemic by working on changing people's mindsets within the company and without, all while attempting to introduce healthier products with lower sugar, fat, and sodium contents.

Now, I was moving to the Vitality Group, part of Discovery Limited, a leading insurance company based in South Africa. I had come to know Vitality over the previous two years because I sat on its US board. It was expanding and wanted me to join full time. Here was yet another iteration of the principle that had inspired and driven me for so long:

public-private partnerships can better people's health more effectively than working toward that goal in isolation. It was what we had done with the international tobacco treaty, for example, and what I had attempted to do by going to PepsiCo and trying to change the culture from within.

I knew that governments were limited in what they could do to encourage people to achieve optimal health. No matter where you are in the world, the law on the books is not the same as the law on the street. For example, declaring that it's illegal to sell tobacco to kids is all well and good, but no one is going to enforce it in a corner store on the south side of Boston or on the streets of Mumbai, where children buy single cigarettes from elderly women sitting on street curbs.

So it is with diet, with governments performing a balancing act between competing interests, from farmers to food companies to consumers. Over the last half-century, in Europe and the United States especially, they have encouraged and subsidized the cultivation of certain crops such as maize and soy, which has kept the price of many foods using these ingredients cheaper than they might otherwise be and has helped stave off famine. But the nutritional value of these food products, which contain ingredients such as high fructose corn syrup, are questionable. Meanwhile, the cost of fresh fruits and vegetables that are vital to our well-being is substantially higher. All of which leads to the question: How do you shift from an agricultural system that sees itself as serving the commercial needs of agriculture rather than the nutritional needs of people?

This is where Vitality comes in, helping to fill the void. It has much to teach us all. Begun in 1992 by South African entrepreneur and actuary Adrian Gore, it was based on the notion that health and life insurance companies should do better than the fusty, reactive model into which they all fit. What would happen, Gore wondered, if a life insurance company started to do what its very name implied it was supposed to do? What would happen if it calculated premiums based on the steps people were taking to improve their health, rather than on a list of exclusions based on their health history? What if it used lower premiums, and other incentives such as cheaper plane tickets, to encourage people to eat better, exercise more, and quit smoking?

What if the life insurance industry was in the business of *promoting* life?

Gore gathered a group of young actuaries to find out. Flipping the bird to conventional insurance wisdom, they turned his experiment into Discovery Limited, the largest private health insurance company in South Africa, and its Vitality-Wellness program of incentives to promote health was the glue that held it all together. Complete with partnerships that involved other companies—supermarkets, gyms, airlines, and even Apple Inc.—to give its members cash-back rebates, cheaper plane tickets, lower premiums, and a watch with fitness-tracking and other health-oriented capabilities, it was revolutionary at the time.

It was the little company that grew and grew. Discovery became South Africa's largest health and automobile insurer, while Vitality, the branch that specialized in life insurance, managed to cut costs and make a profit *because* it was investing in the quality of people's lives and helping them to change their behavior. To join, all people had to do was fill out an online questionnaire, after which they were assigned a "Vitality age" and given a menu of options to lower their risk: eat better, stop smoking, work out more, walk the dog, get regularly screened for medical conditions such as colon and breast cancer, which kill if not caught at an early stage.

To monitor what subscribers did each day and keep a tally of points, Vitality was an early adopter of a twenty-first-century mashup of financial and technical solutions—some wearable, some not. Mindful of privacy concerns, it consulted IT experts as it built firewalls and drafted guidelines to protect from prying eyes the health data collected—including subscribers' employers.

The company's success led to it being enshrined in 2014 as a *Harvard Business Review* case study of what "shared value" partnerships should be.[50] The authors were Dr. Michael Porter, a Harvard economist I first heard speak at the Prague top-to-top meeting and the world's authority on shared value initiatives, and Mark Kramer, a founder and managing director of FSG, a nonprofit consulting firm, who chairs the annual

Shared Value Leadership Summit in New York. They called Vitality the "purest example" of what they were talking about: a business that manages to combine profit with people. It's not about social responsibility, per se, or being green or a good corporate citizen. Instead, it's a new way for companies to achieve economic success—to make profit—through finding a solution to social problems.

It was much like what Indra Nooyi was trying to do at PepsiCo, including going up against shareholders, if necessary.

Like the so-called triple bottom line at pharmaceutical company Novo Nordisk: Planet, People, Profit.

Like providing health insurance through a system that rewards people for treating their bodies and minds with care.

As a passionate advocate of health promotion and disease prevention, as a believer that private enterprise, as long as it is committed, has the power to help change lives for the better, I found Gore's approach impressive and brave. As the founder of the company, his philosophy—to find a balance between profit and people—was hardwired into its very structure. I liked that he measured success by the difference you make to society and the people around you, not by how much money you make. Vitality was born during the apartheid era, when Yasmin and I were still living in Cape Town. At times it was so chaotic, I thought it a miracle that trains continued to run on schedule, that schools held classes, and that hospitals kept their doors open—but somehow, they did. In this maelstrom, Vitality managed to get around and ahead of what was often a clashing mix of old and new government bureaucracies, one failing and the other trying to find its feet.

Fast-forward two decades. It was, as they say, a no-brainer for me to join the company as its senior vice president and executive director of the Vitality Institute. It was as unlike PepsiCo—which had made most of its money in junk food and had not been founded with principles of health in mind— as running shoes are to potato chips.

I'd be working with people who literally put health first, who invested in it, and who were determined to convert a new generation to its simple and dynamic insurance mantra: know your health, improve your health, and enjoy the rewards.

It was a simple message. So simple, in fact, that as I was about to join the company, someone asked me if it had been done before.

"I don't know," I said, "but I'll find out."

Going through US health archives, I discovered that it actually had been done before, more than a hundred years ago. It was an idea that was at once of its time and way, way beyond it— so much so, in fact, that I gave a lecture about it at a business school conference in Chicago in 2016.

Over a century ago, Dr. Irving Fisher, a professor of economics at Yale University and a statistician, inventor, and social campaigner, challenged President Theodore Roosevelt to strike a commission into conserving the health of the American people. Roosevelt was an ardent conservationist (and hunter), known for his protection of the environment, of wild life, public lands, and waterways.

Fisher wanted the president to go further: to look at the conservation of the American people. Didn't they count, too?

Roosevelt agreed that they did. The result was a hundred-page report on the vitality of Americans that called for mass vaccinations against smallpox, the founding of what was called the Life Extension Institute, and the writing of a book, *How to Live—Rules for Healthful Living Based on Modern Science*.[51] In it, Fisher and his colleagues outlined a plan to do something that seemed impossible: extend the average American lifespan from forty-five to sixty years. To achieve that, they dabbled in eugenics—as did many others of that time—recommending that "defectives" be set apart and occasionally, in the worst cases, forcibly sterilized. But the bulk of their work lay in suggesting actions that today may sound like parental advice, but were unheard of back then: Ventilate rooms. Wash hands regularly. Eat lots of fiber. Chew food thoroughly before swallowing, and clean teeth, gums, and tongue afterwards.

Numerous insurance companies, including John Hancock, Metropolitan Life, and Prudential, worked with the institute, using new advertising and public relations techniques to promote healthy behaviors, including pamphlets on healthier living. Policies for the working class were available for weekly premiums that were collected on a door-to-door basis. Lee Frankel, director of MetLife's Welfare Division, introduced methods for collection of new data, such as morbidity statistics, about policyholders.

But it all came crashing down in the 1930s. The American Medical Association successfully sued the institute on the grounds that it was preventing association members from healing the sick by keeping people healthy in the first place.

Plus ça change, plus c'est la même chose, I thought. The more things change, the more they stay the same.

When I came on board in 2011, Vitality was in the midst of worldwide expansion and struggling, because it was concentrating its efforts on workplace environments. Businesses didn't know anything about the company and its philosophy. Why should they offer life insurance to their employees through Vitality instead of a more established, familiar firm such as MetLife Inc. or Prudential Financial Inc?

Soon enough, Gore recognized that trying to launch Vitality as a discrete life and health insurance business in global markets other than the United Kingdom, where it managed to gain a foothold, wasn't going to work. In the United States, Europe, and Asia, it wasn't one of the blue-chip insurance titans but rather an unknown, a baby in a world where constancy, longevity, and tradition reigned. He decided to turn Vitality into a health promotion company that would enter into partnerships with long-established firms such as

Manulife and its US subsidiary, John Hancock Financial Services, and AIA Asia. That way, it would be able to tap into existing, large client bases while remaining faithful to its principles and goals.

My role at the company was broad and difficult to explain. It was the kind of job that could change from one day to the next. It could be about bringing new products into the company and figuring out where they fit, helping to tailor programs for senior citizens or people battling depression, or conducting analytic studies. It could be finding key outside players in business and academia, and expanding the debate between treatment and health promotion. I was a rainmaker and deal maker, the front man who would sit down with people like Arianna Huffington, syndicated columnist and co-founder of the Huffington Post, to talk about the company, and the public health specialist who identified gaps in research and ensured everything we did could be backed up with scientific data. I remained in the United States because the company was in the midst of an international expansion, and we wanted New York City to be our stepping-stone to the rest of the country as well as to Asia and Europe.

Whenever my son asked what I did for a living, I told him: "I actively promote health in all settings so it will benefit us in the long term." It was vague, yet accurate.

As had been my wont in past jobs, I was driven by the rising cost of chronic diseases, including lost productivity in work hours and time spent with family. With the great advances being made in treatment and care, Vitality gave me the chance to look more closely at how a transformation in health promotion and disease prevention can contribute to long-term *and* economic savings and to put my findings into effect.

One of the first people I called for advice was Dr. Don Berwick, who helped shape former president Barack Obama's *Affordable Care Act* and was one of the leaders in US health reform over the past forty years.

"Derek, there are two things you need to know," Berwick said. "The first is that the knowledge-based prevention side of medicine is too weak to fight for itself. And the second is that the voice of the organized private sector in treatment—pharmaceutical companies, hospitals, medical device companies—is all-powerful. They have a huge interest in preserving the way the word 'health' is used. Where are the corporate voices when it comes to prevention?"

His points resonated, for they were the same ones that had been frustrating me ever since I was in medical school back in South Africa—and, as my research uncovered, had been a problem for Fisher's Life Extension Institute.

We scanned the website for the National Institutes of Health (NIH) in an effort to determine what percentage of grant money went to cure disease and what percentage to prevent it. For prevention, including campaigns that promote healthy life habits, the answer was 2 to 6 per cent, a paltry amount no matter how it's spun—but especially when compared to the

94 to 98 per cent dedicated to the search for cures, including clinical interventions and animal experiments.[52]

Our findings helped to reinforce a point I'd been making for years: the size of budget for an area of research is important not only in building a career but also in determining the number of people as a whole going into that field. There aren't many of us to coax people into preventive health careers, or coach them if they make that choice, but there are plenty of people seeking new cures for diseases. We weren't looking to cure cancer; we wanted to prevent it from occurring altogether. For that, we lacked glamor. The public wasn't interested. Insurance companies were supposed to be *boring*.

I understood that it was crucial to foster the development of a new "ecology" of private interests, intertwined with the latest in preventive health innovations. Such innovations were already playing a role in health care in ways that were once unthinkable, heralding a future when chronic diseases such as type 2 diabetes will be better managed in the long term.

Still, in the United States, where obesity was spiraling upward and health care was among the most expensive in the world, I had to figure out a way to heighten our profile. Here, people were—and still are—bombarded twenty-four hours a day with information about the latest trends in diet and exercise and everything in between. The very notion of a health promotion company providing an insurance package sounded flat in comparison to the promise of "Five days to your BEST body ever!"—as if that was possible.

Part of our answer was the creation of the Vitality Institute Commission on Health Promotion and the Prevention of Chronic Disease in Working-Age Americans,[53] launched with great fanfare in May 2013. The aim was twofold: to broaden our profile and ease the way for the company to both globalize its knowledge base and position itself in the vanguard of providing support to global businesses.

We targeted people of working age, because our research found that most of the time, the words "promotion" and "prevention" used together were thought of in connection to children, not adults. We wanted to change that.

We had a veritable who's who from the world of public health involved in the commission. Will Rosenzweig, an entrepreneur, CEO of Physic Ventures, and founder of The Republic of Tea, a specialty company credited with the creation of the premium tea market in the United States, agreed to chair it. Other board members included Ginny Ehrlich, CEO of the Clinton Health Matters Initiative; Susan Dentzer, the senior policy advisor at the Robert Wood Johnson Foundation, the nation's largest philanthropic organization to focus on health and health care; and Clarence Pearson, whom I'd met at WHO when he served as senior advisor to our Department of Aging and Life Course.

Pearson's incredible career spanned sixty years. He was an entrepreneurial global health and management consultant and networker extraordinaire, a raconteur who founded the US National Health Promotion Office in 1941 and was the chief health officer of MetLife in the early 1960s, when the company was doing innovative stuff. He worked with me on the global tobacco control treaty and, when he retired, was the volunteer representative for AARP (American Association of Retired People) at the United Nations and the Council of Foreign Relations. He was an example and a mensch of the highest order.

Pearson died from a rare form of cancer one month before the report was released. I think of him every day. One of the most insightful lessons I ever learned was at a meeting he arranged in Salzburg in the late 1990s.

I was part of a group of youngish professionals beginning to put our stamp on public health policy. We were bedazzled by the presence of Dr. C. Everett Koop, former US surgeon general, and Harlan Cleveland, an American diplomat, educator, and author who served as US ambassador to NATO from 1965 to 1969. I remember Cleveland being asked if he would share the most important principle he'd learned in his illustrious career, and I can hear his simple response as if he was standing right in front of me.

"You have to live with constructive ambiguity," Cleveland said.

"Constructive ambiguity." It became our catchphrase, perfectly describing our experiences in public health as we learned to negotiate around or through political and business roadblocks and fight for what we believed in. We couldn't always expect the world to be pure. The way to make progress was through complicated partnerships, and sometimes we would have to work with our enemies, or at least with people who held different values from our own.

And so the Vitality commission held a series of roundtable meetings across America that highlighted what it means to make markets work for health: that if companies create their goals with health in mind, they can be more profitable, reduce risk, and be of benefit to society. Sometimes, commissioners heard things that ran counter to our beliefs. People described a lack of faith in the insurance industry as a whole: there was an expectation that it would look for the tiniest loophole to get out of paying a benefit. And the future of the labyrinthine, expensive US health care system itself was called into doubt. But we listened. It was a classic example of the process in which we were identifying a social problem and trying to find a way to correct it—a course in twenty-first-century business management that could be called "Shared-Value 101."

The commission's report, published in June 2014, was Vitality's first big achievement. It included a call for more "prevention" science in schools of public health and the NIH, and stressed that in a world of personalized devices—of smartphones, Fitbits, and Apple watches—it is paramount that strong privacy guidelines be implemented and regularly reviewed.[54] With Vitality an early adopter of financial and technical solutions, we were already there. After all, our very business model was based on data from such devices. Following the launch of the company in Germany, an article in *Der Spiegel* magazine wondered how people would feel about the possibility of their employers possessing knowledge about what they do in their private lives. Our answer was: the employers wouldn't know. The data was, and is, secure.[55]

No insurance company had ever gone this consultative route, or taken such a stance in a market-savvy way. The result was that we were seen to be innovative. And complementary to the discourse about prevention and the role industries must play to make markets work: we were trying to push a wide range of companies to define and expand their goals of prevention in ways that would benefit their employees and society as a whole.

Soon Vitality was accepted by leading media, government, corporations, and academics as a go-to place for leadership and insights on adult health promotion, prevention, and workplace health. This, in turn, has led to more doors opening to us, from investors to brokers interested in what we offer and corporations that want to bring us on board.

We helped set the pace and tone by creating partnerships with academic and health organizations, including the Center for Health Incentives and Behavioral Economics at the University of Pennsylvania, where cutting-edge research into behavioral patterns helps to inform public health policy around the world; Harvard University, where we initiated research on the direct and indirect impact of Vitality to help people make positive changes in their lives; and both the Institute for Health Metrics and Evaluation and Truven Health

Analytics, to calculate the health and financial impact of effective preventive measures on the occurrence of noncommunicable diseases and risk-filled behaviors.

Vitality CEO Adrian Gore makes the point beautifully when he says that the insurance sector, as one of only two entities in society (the other being government) to put a monetary value on health, both good and bad, must reduce its costs over time to avoid going bankrupt. "What better way to do that than by *promoting* health?" he asks rhetorically.

That is music to my ears. As was a study by the California-based RAND Corporation, a nonprofit research organization, which used our healthy food discount program in South Africa to show that the rebates do work. Roland Sturm, a senior economist at Rand and study coauthor, noted: "These findings offer good evidence that lowering the cost of nutritionally preferable foods can motivate people to significantly improve their diet. But behavior changes are proportional to price changes. When there is a large gap between people's actual eating behaviors and what nutritionists recommend, even a 25 per cent price change closes just a small fraction of that gap."[56]

We initiated yet another successful study in partnership with experts from the University of Minnesota's Global Landscapes Initiative. Researchers there turned their sights on water and land use patterns for major crops, and proved that shifting to a healthier diet saved 10 per cent of the land used for food production and reduced greenhouse gases.

And yet the commission's recommendations also highlighted gaps in what we were doing at Vitality. Or, more precisely, *not* doing. We emphasized exercise and eating well, but for some reason there was practically no research into alcohol use, mental health, or addiction to prescription medications and tobacco. Think about it: insurers link key sectors of society—food, exercise, and health care. We're the lynchpin that needs to help individual consumers understand how placing a high value on good health will help us all move forward. We were failing utterly.

For example, when the head of the World Economic Forum asked me to chair the Global Agenda Council on Ageing, I realized with a start that one thing I didn't fully support at WHO was the healthy aging program, despite the fact that seniors were among my cluster of responsibilities. Aging and longevity were definitely issues affecting our markets in developing countries, where people were aging faster, and in developed countries such as Singapore, Hong Kong, and right here in the United States. What could we offer them?

I posed the question to staff: "If you're fifty and have lived your life with excess weight and you smoke and so on, what are the best options to extend your life and improve its quality? What happens if you're sixty and in the same position? And what happens if you're isolated and lonely, which we know contribute to disease and death?"

The answers required Vitality's business side to step up and formulate potential plans that would actively support people as they tried to reduce their risk of illness and death—and live better. To reset the prevention agenda, as I wrote in the *American Journal of Preventive Medicine*.[57] In effect, we were saying that it was possible to do a refresh after a half-century or so of hard living, not quite erasing the effects of the past but making the years left better and even adding more good ones.

"Live well and live longer" was the message, not "Be the best you can in the time you have left."

It's a program that encompasses a future where people will live longer than ever before. As hard as it may be for my teenaged son and his peers to imagine, advances in health care and prevention indicate that fully half of them will live to be at least one hundred years old. When they reach the age of fifty, it won't be such a milestone any longer, but simply the start of the second half of their lives.

But when it came to tobacco, the old nemesis that I had been battling against ever since university, we had the biggest problem of all. Really, the only counsel we gave members who were trying to quit was to consult a 1985 book called *The Easy Way to Stop Smoking* and look into its affiliated online and in-person seminars and counselling programs. The author, Allen Carr, was a British accountant turned self-help guru who also penned *Easy Way* books about stopping drinking and weight loss. He claimed he managed to quit smoking one hundred cigarettes a day when he was in his late forties after he had the epiphany that nicotine turned him into an addict. As long as he recognized it was withdrawal that was making him feel "empty and insecure," it was easy to find the strength of will not to take up smoking again.

"I was a serial quitter," he wrote in the 280-page book, which is probably 279 pages too long in its attempt to explain a strange feat of mental gymnastics to readers. "I once lasted six months of sheer hell before I caved in and lit one up."

Carr, who died of lung cancer in 2006, recommended that if you really wanted to quit smoking, forget nicotine replacements such as gum or the patch. Just quit, and whenever you think about having a cigarette, ask yourself: "Do I want to become a smoker again, all day, every day sticking those things into my mouth, setting light to them, never being allowed to stop?"[58]

To me, it sounded lame at best, a huckster's approach at worst, and pretty well near damned impossible to accomplish in the long term. Where, I wondered, was the evidence that it worked? As hard as I tried, the only study I managed to unearth that said *some* good things about Carr's method was an obscure Austrian-German paper that contained anecdotal evidence. Now stories may be very nice, but they are most definitely not the basis on which to introduce and implement policy. No one is going to say, "Hey, use this statin drug to lower your cholesterol and prevent heart attacks and strokes because we heard it works!" Instead, it takes years of hard, scientific research, including several phases of study and in-depth reports, before a drug is allowed to be sold on the market.

I needed to find something else—a proven program, a therapy, a reduced-risk tobacco replacement—that we could provide Vitality members and that would be of shared value, helping to solve the problem while benefiting us, too. But where to start?

In 2015, I was putting my thoughts to paper when the Vitality UK team approached me to say the health editor at *The Spectator* wanted an op-ed piece about tobacco products and harm reduction. Would I write it?

"Absolutely," I said.

First, I reviewed what we had at WHO in the buildup to the global tobacco control treaty. More precisely, I reviewed what evidence had been ignored, unwittingly or not. Sure enough, we had missed data about a product called snus, which may have helped us back then in our effort to lower the rate of tobacco-caused diseases and death.

Snus is a moist, air-dried tobacco that has been declared illegal in every EU country save Sweden. It is also legal in Norway, which is not a member of the European Union. At WHO, it had been dismissed as just another form of dirty chewing tobacco, much like the kind professional baseball players in the United States still use despite a league ban. Beyond resulting in disgusting gobs of brown spit, the players have a heightened risk of mouth, tongue, cheek, and throat cancers. The statistics for snus, however, told another story: the smoking rate in Sweden was the lowest in the European Union, and snus appeared to play a major role in that achievement, given that 54 per cent of its users were ex-smokers, most of them men.[59]

An independent overview in a 2008 issue of *The Lancet Oncology* summarized the findings of three studies, two from Sweden and one from Norway.[60] They concluded that snus, which is usually placed inside the upper lip and from there nicotine is released into the body, posed little to no increased risk of oral cancer over other nicotine replacement therapies. Also, a 2008 report by EU scientists found that, while all smokeless products caused oral lesions and had some level of health risk, as a whole, they were substantially less hazardous than cigarettes.[61]

When I considered that more Swedish men than women used snus, at 20 per cent compared to 2 per cent,[62] and that Swedish men had the lowest death rate of any group anywhere in the European Union,[63] my thinking about the product changed. To the point that I wondered why there was such resistance to making it legal. Nothing is ever 100 per cent safe, be it coffee, chocolate, or walking across a street. But the evidence here indicated that snus was harm reducing. It was working. Given the studies I was reading, could the same argument be applied to the emerging market of e-cigs? Was it fair for regulatory bodies around the world to treat them as if they were cigarettes? I didn't think so.

There you are, about to get into trouble again, doing the unthinkable by questioning what you once treated as gospel, I thought to myself.

The Spectator op-ed piece was published on February 21, 2015, under the provocative headline, "E-cigarettes save lives." The sub-headline was equally provocative: "I understand why anti-smoking activists so mistrust vaping. I'm one of them. But the evidence is clear."[64]

I wrote that it's not surprising most people in the public health sphere echo the position of Dr. Neil Schluger, a lung specialist and medical professor at Columbia University. "If there ever was an industry that does not deserve the benefit of the doubt when it comes to protecting or promoting the public's health, it is the tobacco industry," he has said. After all, their deceptions included any number of lies about the deadly effects of tar and other chemicals in combustible cigarettes and the development and misleading marketing of so-called low-tar products, which they claimed caused less harm when the opposite was true. It was only natural that electronic cigarettes would be cast as the industry's latest ruse, right? But after reading and researching, it seemed to me that wasn't the case at all.

I noted that the statistics were (and still are) appalling. That even though I harp on the numbers all the time, each time I do, they make me shiver in horror: 1.3 billion smokers in the world and roughly 6 million smoking-related deaths each year. Six *million*. In the United Kingdom alone, there are 80,000 deaths each year due to smoking, which accounts for 18 per cent of all deaths there on an annual basis. And for every death, there are more than 20 more smokers who suffer from tobacco-related diseases, which result in 450,000 hospital admissions each year.

I argued that even though traditionalists demand more of the same policies outlined in the WHO tobacco treaty that have already significantly reduced tobacco use—excise taxes, smoke-free workplaces, and more effective anti-smoking advertising—such a one-size-fits-all approach to tobacco control is doomed to fail. In the United States, for example, long-term projections state that these kinds of measures would reduce smoking from the current 15 per cent to 10 per cent by the year 2030. That still leaves millions of smokers at risk—millions who may benefit by taking up e-cigarettes.

Calling for higher excise taxes, I wrote, ignores rising concerns about their regressive impact on poorer and more-addicted smokers. Furthermore, advances in the genetics of nicotine use suggest that no matter the cost, half of all smokers don't have a choice because they are so addicted to nicotine. According to the United Kingdom's Action on Smoking and Health, about 2.8 million British adults currently use e-cigarettes—38 per cent claimed the e-cigs helped them stop smoking entirely and 22 per cent said they helped them reduce the number of cigarettes they smoke. And I noted that Robert West, a professor of health psychology at University College London, reported that e-cig use by people who have never smoked before is negligible.

I addressed safety concerns, referring to two British analyses that reviewed toxicological, laboratory, and clinical research on

the potential risks of e-cigs. The conclusion was that they are
by far less harmful than smoking, and that "significant health
benefits are expected in smokers who switch from tobacco
to e-cigs." Yet governments around the world, public health
agencies, and WHO remained unconvinced and continued to
treat e-cigs as if they were cigarettes containing tobacco. There
was no such thing as a safe cigarette, they maintained. What
if kids start to use them, they worried. Or pregnant women?

There was deep distrust of tobacco companies—a distrust
I had always shared—and a reluctance to deal with them
in any way other than as an enemy that must be monitored
and regulated. I understood why they were claiming there
is no safe cigarette. I could understand why there was worry
about non-toxic nanoparticles being inhaled deep into the
lungs and embedded in the alveoli, leading or contributing
to asthma and other conditions. But in the greater scheme of
things, it was necessary to think the unthinkable. To keep an
open mind.

To remember: e-cigs don't contain tar.

I concluded *The Spectator* piece with this: "At the moment,
it's estimated that there will be a billion tobacco-related
deaths before 2100. That is a dreadful prospect. E-cigs and
other nicotine-delivery devices such as vaping pipes offer us
the chance to reduce that total. All of us involved in tobacco
control need to keep that prize in mind as we redouble efforts
to make up for 50 years of ignoring the simple reality that
smoking kills and nicotine does not."

Reaction was immediate. It became the most downloaded article in the history of *The Spectator*'s online health section. All of a sudden, I was the darling of the e-cig world—the public health expert, the antitobacco crusader, an architect of WHO's global tobacco control treaty who changed his mind. I fielded calls and e-mails from journalists, outraged former colleagues, and e-cig lobbyists who were happy to have an ally. I heard from David Graham, an old friend from the pharmaceutical industry with an expertise in nicotine replacement therapy; after stints in executive positions at Pharmacia & Upjohn and Johnson & Johnson, he'd gone to Pfizer and created a global advisory board for nicotine cessation on which I sat. But it didn't go anywhere, and the last I'd heard, he was heading external relations for a boutique American e-cig firm called NJOY, which was the first company to make the product in the United States. He'd become impatient with Johnson & Johnson, which had the licence to manufacture Nicorette Gum but wasn't moving fast enough, as far as he was concerned.

"No big company wants to manufacture a product that looks like a cigarette," he complained to me. "There's no understanding of the intimate behaviour of a smoker."

I agreed, and arranged for Vitality to conduct a large long-term clinical trial into the use of e-cigs with six thousand of our members. It is being done now in conjunction with the Center for Health Incentives and Behavioral Economics at the University of Pennsylvania. Preliminary findings are expected sometime in 2018.

I gave speeches and interviews and I participated in debates. Then, on May 5, 2015, not quite three months after the op-ed piece turned me into a lightning rod for both sides—and ten years since I had last spoken to her when I was at Yale—I got an e-mail from the lawyer I had first encountered years earlier during the WHO tobacco control hearing. She had been the BAT representative. Now working for Philip Morris International, she wrote that tobacco companies still need to do a lot to rectify past wrongs and that a public statement on their intention to change should be backed up by real, drastic action.

"But it's only going to be PMI that will do that, and then the others will follow," she continued. "Perhaps it would be good timing to talk about this. Would you be prepared to have a chat with me and a couple of senior people from PMI to take this forward? They want to do something but don't know what to do. I told them what to do, but who am I to tell them? If they heard it from you it might just happen!"

Even though she knew it seemed a bit like déjà vu, given my previous meeting with BAT executives a decade earlier, she said there was real will at PMI to change. "We could do something big!" she concluded.

At the time, I had little inkling just how big that something would be.

10

IN THE LAIR OF THE ENEMY

September 2015, Geneva Airport: As I disembarked the plane, for one moment I wished I had worn a hat with a wide brim that I could pull down over my brow. The customs agent asked no questions before stamping my passport. With no checked baggage, I cautiously made my way into the arrivals area, my eyes darting left and right to see if there was anyone I knew. There was no one. Relieved, I spotted a driver in a plain dark suit standing with a sign that said, simply, "PMI."

Here we go, I thought.

For me, the thirty-seven-mile drive along the A1 highway to the Beau-Rivage Palace hotel on the shores of Lake Geneva in Lausanne was a trip down memory lane. I had traveled this route hundreds, maybe thousands, of times before, past the picturesque towns of Versoix, Coppet, and Nyon, where Yasmin and I lived for nearly nine years, where our son was conceived.

The lake streaked by, blue, black, and green in the early autumn light, familiar and foreign at the same time. I thought of all the steps, twists, and turns that got me here. Of the public hearings that WHO held in the buildup for the tobacco control treaty and of the Scotch- and shoe-loving lawyer who was there every day for BAT—as far as I was concerned, the only one of their representatives who tried to keep an open mind and really understand what was going on.

After her May 5 e-mail to me, we'd arranged to meet the following week for breakfast in London, England. I would be attending a health committee meeting of the Wellcome Trust, the world's largest medical charity that funds research into human and animal health. I remembered perfectly what I ate: scrambled eggs, smoked salmon, fresh-squeezed carrot juice, and a cappuccino. She had Earl Grey tea and cut right to the chase.

"PMI is committed to producing lower-risk tobacco products, and they're willing to send representatives to you in Connecticut to describe what they're doing. Afterwards, if you think what they say has merit, then we want you to come to Lausanne, visit The Cube to see for yourself, and possibly meet the CEO."

My heart sank. Without saying it out loud, I suspected what she wanted. PMI would not want to convene a meeting so that the CEO and I could simply sit down and shoot the breeze about nothing. "The Cube" is PMI's twinkling glass crucible for research and development in Neuchâtel, France, and I would be a high-profile catch, an outspoken enemy of everything the company represented finally brought on side. Some would undoubtedly call it a sellout and claim that big money had brought me to heel; a reverse Marlboro Man for the ages, this time one who never smoked and is so oriented toward health, his Twitter handle is @swimdaily. Still, I had nothing to lose by receiving PMI representatives on my home turf in Connecticut. It would be like meeting all those multinational food company executives all those years ago back in the village of Échenevex, surrounded by fields and cows. Even better, I would be in my comfort zone, able to control what happens—and if I didn't like what they had to say, then I could just get up, get into my car, and drive off.

I said: "Sure."

It happened fast. By the end of May, an economist with expertise in health issues, who is now PMI's vice president of strategic policy initiatives, and the company's director of global policy and advocacy were in Southport. We met in a hotel down the street from my home, chitchatting before going upstairs to a room so I could review the research for myself. The economist had been a nonsmoker all his life, a man who was clearly inspired by PMI's new mantra. The director of global policy was more flamboyant, a guy who needed a nicotine dose every few minutes and smoked a prototype of IQOS, PMI's smokeless "heat-not-burn" hybrid between analogs and e-cigs, with a name that is an acronym for "I Quit Ordinary Smoking." Marketed to smokers who crave the taste of real cigarettes, it looks like a classic Marlboro cigarette and contains real tobacco refills. But rather than burn the tobacco, which produces the carcinogenic smoke and tar, it heats it to create a tobacco-flavored vapor. The novel idea behind it is that heating tobacco reduces or eliminates the formation of many of the deadly compounds produced at the high temperatures needed for combustion.

They were a tag team, the two of them, fast talking, a bit nervous but prepared with an in-depth presentation: molecular biology reports on risk measurement and reduction, lots of photos and videos of shiny new machinery, experiments that mimicked the rhythmic movement of cilia in the lungs as they worked to keep the airways free of mucus and dirt. The information kept coming, showing enough to convince me they were serious about what they were doing—and make me want more.

"And we're not just investing in the research and science," they told me. "The *whole* company is invested in this change."

I'd heard that before. I asked: "What's your long-term strategy?"

The answer was so unexpected it nearly knocked me over. "We want you to join us in some way on a long-term journey to make cigarettes obsolete."

I thought, *What a difference from the presentations about reduced risk tobacco products I first heard during the tobacco treaty hearings at WHO.*

And: *Are they serious?*

All sorts of questions swirled through my mind. What would I tell Vitality? How would my colleagues respond if I told them that I had met with PMI executives? That I wanted our company to work with PMI in some capacity because they wanted people to smoke fewer cigarettes, too? That I might be consultant to that process? And would I be guilty of doing what, in the past, we accused others of doing: working with an enemy, sucked in by a line and some research? Of being co-opted? Would Vitality feel the need to keep such co-operation a secret? Did *I* feel the need for that? Could an insurance business built on the premise of promoting life and rewarding positive health initiatives ever work with a tobacco company, openly or not? Who would support me if I crossed that line? I'd have to explain to my colleagues, my friends, my siblings, and my son.

I imagined myself saying: Julian, your dad, who has spent his life campaigning against smoking, has a contract to consult for one of the biggest tobacco companies in the world.

How would *that* go over?

If I thought that the criticism and contempt I endured when I went to work for PepsiCo or when I wrote the op-ed piece in *The Spectator* was bad, this would be ten times, one hundred times, a thousand million times worse.

The Spectator piece was but one man's opinion; readers could keep it for reference or use it to line their kitty litter box. PepsiCo and other multinationals might be disliked, but they make products like hummus and oatmeal that mitigate their badness. The tobacco companies were hated. I'd hated them. They were the enemy. The cause of horrible diseases and countless deaths. That's why this was totally, absolutely unthinkable. Impossible. And yet, I'd already come out in public about supporting e-cigarettes, because I believed they would help save millions of lives in the future that would otherwise be lost to cancer, chronic obstructive pulmonary disease, and other tobacco-related conditions.

I could see other arguments, too. The suspicions. The optics of PMI—the biggest of Big Tobacco—with its built-in market of addicts, wanting to break into a business begun by smaller boutique companies such as NJOY, which, by the way, didn't carry the baggage of having spent the past who-knew-how-many generations knowingly killing people and lying about it.

The conversation in my mind went something like this:

What's in it for them? Is it because they want to make amends for their actions in the past? Do they see a new avenue to make profits? Or is it a bit of both?

Does it matter? There are billions of smokers around the world and more who will take up the habit in the future. If we can help save, say, half of them, by getting them to switch, that's a good thing, right?

Right. (That said with a silent little snicker.)

You've already taken it on the chin at PepsiCo. That was nothing. This would be a marathon—no, a swimming ultra-marathon in a river filled with piranha, poisonous spiders, and tiger fish with razor-sharp teeth.

But you're nothing if not pragmatic—and you're a very good swimmer.

When the two men invited me to visit them in Switzerland and France, I said: "In principle, I accept your offer—but I need to speak with my wife."

Yasmin had been my moral barometer ever since we were at the University of Cape Town together. Now, she was calm and realistic. "Go," she said. "See what they're doing but tell no one, not colleagues and definitely not the media."

She understood immediately the absolute simplicity of the argument for e-cigs: if you eliminate tar, you greatly reduce the risk. I'd been telling her for ages and we'd been married long enough that she could anticipate what was going to come out of my mouth before I did. And what did I have to lose?

■

The PMI driver was pulling the limo up to the white-painted brick front of the Beau-Rivage hotel, with the lake twinkling on the other side.

"I need to swim," I said to no one in particular.

And so, the ultramarathon began.

The meeting with André Calantzopoulos, the CEO, was scheduled for noon on the day I arrived and was expected to last no longer than thirty minutes. It was supposed to be perfunctory, little more than "hello and nice to meet you." Afterwards, the health economist, the director of global policy, and the lawyer, without whom I wouldn't have been here in the first place, were to escort me to The Cube to see the labs and review more research. I did laps in the hotel pool for forty minutes, showered, dressed, and went for a long walk along the lake, pulling up the collar of my coat against the wind. It was chilly and the few leaves left on the trees wouldn't be there for long. Walking gave me a chance to have a last conversation between doubtful me and curious me, and maybe a bit of a pep talk.

Am I doing the right thing? I asked myself yet again.

I'm doing what needs to be done, came the answer. I've done that all my life. I take risks in the name of the greater good, and I don't always tread down the conventional path.

Echoing in my head was the word of caution once offered to me by Timothy Stamps, the former minister of health in Zimbabwe, as we surreptitiously planned the first-ever all-Africa conference on tobacco control back in the early '90s. I had asked how we could ever possibly work with Big Tobacco and tobacco growers. "When you sup with the devil, Derek, make sure you use a spoon with a long handle," he said in his clipped British accent. I felt a great hole open up in me when he died on November 26, 2017, only five days after Zimbabwe's strongman president Robert Mugabe was forced from office. And the image of supping with the devil from as far away as possible has stayed with me when meeting groups with whom I don't feel comfortable.

Do the means justify the end? Or, better, does the end justify the means?

"Challenge," I instructed myself out loud. "Listen before asking questions and call them on it if you sense they're giving you a cynical line. They want you here. You don't need them. Go in with a long-handled spoon."

The director of global policy picked me up at the hotel. He seemed nervous, like an actor on the opening night of a show as the curtain is about to be pulled back. In contrast, I felt no hint of nerves. The swim and walk helped calm me.

We pulled up in front of PMI's modern stone and glass headquarters. Directly across the street sits BAT's headquarters, inscrutable in daylight with windows I couldn't see through.

I thought: *How ironic.*

Walking into Calantzopoulos's office, I first saw some Ferrari model race cars set out on a table. It turned out he's passionate about the car and owns six or seven real ones. To break the ice—and, in general, having no idea how to speak to people who are crazy about cars—I asked: "What colors do they come in?"

"Red," he replied. "It's the color of Ferrari."

Everything about him was contained. Curly hair cut short. A slim build in a perfectly tailored suit. A strong handshake, dark eyes that observed without giving away his thoughts. Of Greek heritage, he was a design engineer in the automotive industry before joining PMI. As we chatted politely, it turned out my in-laws had a home on the same little-known island in the Aegean Sea that he visited all the time, Alonissos.

True, we were establishing common ground. Still, it felt awkward, which was to be expected in a meeting between two people who have spent much of their professional lives on opposite sides of the playing field.

We drank espressos in little ceramic cups. Throughout, like the company's director of global policy, he chain-smoked IQOSs. They seemed a part of him. He reminded me of my-mother-and-her-cigarette, never one without the other.

We talked about my background and how I perceived tobacco companies. About the fundamental mistrust I had had for years because of the lies they told, the lengths to which they went to misrepresent the science and the deathly danger posed by the products.

"It wasn't easy coming here, I'm sure," he said. "But I've been here long enough to believe we now have the technological capability to make real changes. To make combustible cigarettes a relic of the past. I have daughters and I don't want them to smoke. You understand."

I thought of the chart I was shown at BAT back in 2005 that highlighted the huge sales gap between tobacco and reduced-risk products. "How do you plan to adjust the markets?" I asked.

"A few years ago, we saw this coming and invested several billions of dollars into our research facility," he replied. "The results have been beyond our expectations. What we have to figure out is how to bridge the divide between accessibility in the public sphere and the product, given our history."

He paused. Then asked, "What would it take for us to do it?"

I was thrust back to my lunch with Nooyi at PepsiCo, when she told me she wanted the company to become the healthiest in the world and asked pretty much the same question. I had no easy answer then or now. *Especially* now, sitting across from a man who the bulk of the health community would consider Public Enemy No. 1.

But I was ready for this question and gave it a go, reciting from a list of conditions I had memorized.

"You have to make a public statement that combustible tobacco will be obsolete by a certain definite date," I said.

And: "You have to stop underhanded lobbying for things such as lower excise taxes."

And: "Stop fighting legislation around the world, and pull back on lawsuits."

And: "You have to establish a fund to ensure sustainability."

And: "You have to link compensation for company executives around the world to positive changes in your product portfolio."

And: "You have to make sure that your marketing, production, and R & D divisions are all in sync. My experience at PepsiCo was that R & D did a great job of developing new products, yet most of them didn't have a chance in hell of seeing the light of day."

Although Calantzopoulos didn't give an unqualified "yes" to each demand, he didn't say "no," either. I was pleasantly surprised when he offered a few possible conditions of his own, including licensing in the public domain some of the scientific innovations PMI researchers had come up with.

"Why should we keep it to ourselves when we can improve the safety of the products?" he asked.

I was impressed and agreed to further discussions over the next few months. Maybe PMI's lawyer was right. Maybe the company really was ready to change. But first, I needed to see if Calantzopoulos fulfilled, or at least tried to fulfill, the conditions I'd set out for him and the company. They wouldn't be easy, but for me, they were a necessary first step.

By the time we finished talking and looked at our watches, we were startled to see that two hours had passed. When I left his office, the health economist, the director of global policy, and the lawyer were still waiting in the anteroom, anxious and pacing. Indeed, the director, who'd been nervous enough when he picked me up at the hotel, now looked like he was about to jump out of his skin.

"What happened?" they asked.

"We had a full and frank discussion," I said.

"And?" they prompted.

"Let's wait and see."

The curtain had risen on the play, even with the script still a work in progress. It felt like I was caught in a whirlwind, only I wasn't sure if it was going to take me up or knock me down.

■

The three PMI executives took me to The Cube, where I was shown the laboratories and spoke with the company's scientists. They all had similar stories: they had come from companies such as Novartis and Johnson & Johnson because they believed in the science and what they were doing. To my eyes, PMI's investment was obvious and serious. I had never before seen such research in my life, down to the intricate model of a trachea and lungs, complete with cilia, bronchi, bronchioles, and alveoli. The idea was to measure the effect of the nicotine vapor on the lungs.

Was I being wooed? Probably a bit. But I couldn't help being impressed—and with the knowledge I had gathered while writing my opinion piece for *The Spectator* in early 2015, I recognized that even if I was the object of a public relations charm offensive, it didn't much matter. I was fascinated and excited by what was happening in the field.

As an epidemiologist with a mother who had been a recalcitrant smoker for most of her life, and with aunts and other relatives who died of tobacco-related causes, I knew what addiction looked like. Even though I knew I would campaign against combustible cigarettes until such time as I was on my own deathbed, it was brought home to me that millions upon millions of lives could be saved if products such as e-cigarettes and IQOS were readily available on the market. And even though their long-term health effects wouldn't be known for years hence, I thought I was willing to take the chance.

The situation certainly can't get any worse than it is right now, I thought.

It was the pragmatist in me, and the South African who grew up and worked for change from within a repressive, racist regime because I knew that change would inexorably come. And I wished I had been able to save my relatives who died in such grisly, gasping ways.

■

This is what I know: change takes time, and changing an industry is best done in baby steps. That's progress. No matter my job, I have never expected everything and everyone to fall in line on my say-so or because it's the best thing to do. Things fall apart and get put back together. People fall down and get back up. As do I, because I believe in saving lives—and because I have to believe that Calantzopoulos and PMI are committed to that, too. Some call me naive. Some call me a sellout. And some suggest that people who play nice with tobacco companies risk playing the role of the frog who agrees to carry a scorpion across a stream on his back, only to have the scorpion sting him when they're halfway across.

"Why?" the frog asks as they both begin to drown.

"It's my nature," the scorpion says.

I have always worked to improve public health and heighten prevention, no matter what it takes. To that end, I take calculated risks, as the actuaries at Vitality would say. When I went back to them with the news that I'd talked with the CEO of PMI and would continue to do so, it was no surprise that they were worried about how such meetings would look to others. I was, too. But they were interested in the science, and in PMI's commitment to change and to leading the way for other companies to change, too.

Maybe it's Calantzopoulos's daughters who drive him. Maybe he's a good man who wants to help solve a grievous social problem or maybe he just sees the writing on the wall. The thing is, his reasons don't matter. His actions do. And so far, he has proved he is a man of action and remains true to his word.

In August 2016, at an annual international trade meeting he went public with his intention to make cigarettes a thing of the past, a statement that wasn't covered in the media because there were few journalists present. He reiterated that undertaking in a much more public fashion three months later, when the company finally launched IQOS.

"I believe that there will come a moment in time where we have sufficient adoption of this alternative product and sufficient awareness to start envisaging—together with governments—a phase-out period for cigarettes," he told BBC Radio 4's *Today* program. "I hope this time will come soon."[65]

In the spring of 2017, he was in Dubai to host PMI's first transformation meeting, with board members, executives from every country the company does business in—and me. It was clear that people at PMI had accepted that this big change was happening. There was not one question about whether or not it was possible, or why their CEO insisted on doing it in the first place. Instead, questions revolved around the nuts and bolts of transformation: for example, how to transform a huge cigarette factory in Turkey into an IQOS hub, and what form new marketing will take.

To further demonstrate his commitment, Calantzopoulos managed to convince a UK-based corporate consultant company known for choosing its clients carefully and helping them define principles and goals that make them better corporate citizens to accept PMI as a client. Also in the spring of 2017, PMI's website went live with its commitment, announcing a smoke-free future on its home page and asking visitors to click through to its manifesto: "Designing a Smoke-Free Future."

"In changing times," it says, "you can always choose to do nothing. Instead, we've set a new course for the company. We've chosen to do something really big."

The plan set out is a classic shared-value case as outlined by Porter and Kramer. Develop, market, and sell smoke-free products; transition to only dealing in smoke-free products; propose regulatory policies that encourage use of smoke-free products in place of tobacco; implement world-class sustainability throughout the company; attract the best international talent; be transparent; and provide superior returns for shareholders.[66]

People will scoff. Of *course* they will! How, they will ask, can a behemoth that has lied for so long while pushing its tobacco products, despite incontrovertible evidence that they cause users to get sick and die, be part of the solution? It's a fair question, and I'm not sure if there is a definitive answer. Sometimes, you just have to trust your feelings and what is right there before your eyes. It won't happen overnight. It never does. But I believe it will be easier for PMI, which has always marketed one product, to transform itself than it has been for PepsiCo, with the myriad goods it offers. Having seen the seriousness and dedication first-hand in every part of PMI, I think its progress has already surpassed that of PepsiCo and that a few years down the road, it will be eons ahead. With that in mind, I've taken the next step, too. It's a major one.

I've left Vitality and gone to work with PMI full-time as first-ever chair of its grandly named Foundation for a Smoke-Free World. There. I've said it in black and white, with all the shades of gray in between.

I suspected the job offer was coming. I knew that PMI was drawing up a draft charter and governance guidelines that would be legally constituted as a Swiss foundation with a funding mechanism and advisory committees. I knew it was being established to support the company as it embarked on a full-scale effort to ensure that reduced-risk products replace combustible cigarettes to the benefit of smokers, society, the company, and the shareholders. The six pages outlined in detail PMI's commitment to this undertaking, and reflected every condition I set out in my first conversation with Calantzopoulos that September afternoon in 2015.

When he approached me with the draft in hand and a look of uncertainty in his eyes, and asked me to lead the effort, I gulped and said, "Yes."

Unspoken were the sentiments I'd felt on that plane trip to Geneva for our first meeting. *What* was I doing? How would it be seen in a world that distrusts tobacco companies?

When I said "yes" to the job with the foundation, I realized that I couldn't continue for Vitality, at least not for long. It was paramount that I avoid conflicts of interest and any appearance of conflict of interest. I didn't want someone at one of the insurance companies we have partnered with around the world to question the wisdom of my working simultaneously for both—or, more probably, question my sanity altogether. To be honest, sometimes I question it, too. But when I do, I remind myself that I'm entering a world where I can help make great changes, which has been a driving force ever since I entered medical school. I tell myself that the risk is worth it, that life is full of risks and if you don't take them, you will end up standing still and doing nothing. Be it swimming from Cape Town to Robben Island, working in the South African townships amid rioting, fighting for a tobacco control treaty in the face of harsh and sneakily subversive opposition, trying to change PepsiCo's culture from within, I've always tried to make a difference in a positive way. Why not here, with PMI?

Call me deluded, a dreamer, or a pragmatist, but for me, the statistics tell a stark story: if you use these products, you are between 80 and 95 per cent less likely to contract a tobacco-related disease.[67] Certainly, quitting smoking altogether is the gold standard against which everything else must be measured. At the same time, one of every two smokers will get sick. That is the hard truth. They will contract lung cancer, or heart disease, or a chronic obstructive pulmonary condition such as emphysema. Each time they put a lit cigarette to their lips and take a drag, they're taking a gamble, and even if they get away with it in the short term, one way or another, the house will always win.

I want to help change those odds.

11

BATTLE POSITIONS!

The last paper I helped work on for Vitality, published in late June 2017 in the *Harvard Business Review*, was entitled "Can Insurance Companies Incentivize Their Customers to Be Healthier?"[68] Substitute "Tobacco" for "Insurance" and, as jarring and counterintuitive as it may sound, it could very well be a treatise on what we are trying to accomplish at PMI.

The paper starts with the presumption, shared by behavioral economists, that the power of instant gratification and wishful thinking all too often lead to poor decisions. Like reaching for that last slice of cake or skipping a workout because it can get done "later." "The behavioral biases play out in a simple paradox," it stated. "People over-consume health care but under-consume prevention, and insurers or taxpayers are left with the bill. The same plays out with many lines of insurance, where the immediate benefits of poor choices outweigh the often-hidden cost of dealing with their consequences, such as reckless driving or failing to flood-proof infrastructure in highly exposed communities."

Why not think of e-cigarettes and IQOS products as preventive, too?

I knew that some people would consider that contention nothing less than blasphemy because such products are all too often considered as dangerous, if not more, than those products that contain tobacco and other carcinogens. Thus, I braced myself—even more than I'd had to when joining PepsiCo—to absorb and counter their hostility and wrath. I knew it would be of no use whatsoever to try to talk to some of them. People like Dr. Vera da Costa e Silva, a former colleague who now heads WHO's secretariat for the global tobacco control treaty; Dr. Stanton Glantz, the Truth Initiative Distinguished Professor of Tobacco Control at the University of California, San Francisco; and Matthew Myers, who heads an NGO called Campaign for Tobacco-Free Kids. Without a doubt, they would consider me a traitor no matter what I said or what studies I presented. It wouldn't help for me to show them data indicating that the bulk of users are not new smokers at all or to provide evidence that governments and companies are working together to dampen down the allure of such products by ensuring there is no glamor involved, no cool flavors, and no colored vapor. It would be for naught for me to point out strict policies about the minimum age to purchase, limits on advertising, and tamperproof packaging able to withstand repeated attempts by children to open it. Or point out the sad fact that people will smoke, no matter the health consequences. That is the nature of life—and death. Teens will smoke, too. It is in their makeup to rebel and try out new things, despite lectures about the risks in the short, and especially long, term.

It would all fall on deaf ears, as would the assurances that Philip Morris International is not out to ensnare a new group of young smokers and that its goal is to eradicate combustible cigarettes from its portfolio in the future. To those people, I have simply gone over to the dark side, a former ally turned traitor and foe.

There have been suspicions and suggestions that I have become a shill for the company. A mouthpiece being paid lots of money. A sellout. But I am not. I believe in the science. In the hard evidence before me. And right now, according to numerous British and American studies, the evidence is clear: the smoking rate among kids is at an all-time low. Has that coincided with an uptick in the use of e-cigs over the last five or six years? Yes, but when you factor in that they're smoking fewer cigarettes altogether, it just proves that kids will be kids. They don't yet have the sense of mortality that will inevitably come. They experiment and they try to push the limits. Isn't it a good thing that they are pushing those limits with a product that is, according to the available data, much less deadly than the alternative? That point is why I have a problem with a report published in December 2016 by the US Office of the Surgeon General about e-cigarette use in young people. In its call for the government to regulate the sale of e-cigs, the report failed to note the dramatic difference in risk between smoking combustible cigarettes and the alternative.

As for fears that this is but a trick by the tobacco industry to cement its position in a changing market, with profit as its sole driver? Over the course of my professional life, I have learned that there doesn't have to be an inherent conflict between profit and health. As a student, I may have started out believing that, but through experience, I've come to learn that the best way—the *only* way—to effect real, lasting change is through partnerships. As the saying goes, sometimes you have to dance with the one who "brung" you, and right now, PMI is leading the way.

In an effort to cut into our market, there already has been an increase in the marketing of smoking cessation products such as nicotine gum and the patch, which is fine in and of itself. But studies show they are not as effective as e-cigarettes and IQOS in helping people to quit smoking.

In the twelve months from April 2016 to March 2017, the market for IQOS in Japan increased from a 1.6 per cent market share to an astounding 10 per cent, indicating the product is more than catching on. In the last three years alone, more than two million adult smokers in twenty-five markets around the world have quit cigarettes for the new product. PMI plans to meet global demand by doubling the production of heat-not-burn products to one hundred billion by the end of 2018, well on its way to effectively becoming the third-largest brand in the world, save for China and just behind Marlboro and Winston.

Change is coming. Some of it is already here.

There are challenges ahead on several fronts, but they all come down to one important distinction: e-cigs and PMI's heat-not-burn products are not the same as combustible cigarettes. Breathe in a lungful of cigarette smoke and you're breathing in tar and toxic chemicals like tobacco-specific nitrosamines, all of which turn lungs from a healthy pink to black. Breathe in the vapor from an e-cig or IQOS and that doesn't happen. Period. That said, what does happen in users is up for debate right now; for example, whether or not nanoparticles lodge deep in the lungs' lining and possibly cause or exacerbate conditions such as asthma or diabetes, or have adverse effects on the fetus of a pregnant woman. And frankly, in the case of pregnant women, they should avoid a lot of things to keep their fetuses healthy, from alcohol to smoking and even high-impact exercise.

■

Since my op-ed article in *The Spectator* about e-cigarettes, there have been more studies about the effects of such products that help bolster my position and that of Public Health

England. This includes an independent two-hundred-page report by the United Kingdom's Royal College of Physicians that distilled the results of dozens of studies that examined the science, public policy, regulation, and ethics surrounding e-cigarettes and other non-tobacco sources of nicotine. Published in April 2016, it concluded that, contrary to public fears, e-cigarettes are not a gateway to smoking but, rather, were limited to those who already use, or have used, tobacco, and that using them can be an important step for hard-core smokers to take before trying to quit the habit altogether.[69] The report acknowledged that the effects from long-term use of e-cigarettes won't be known until years from now because they are so new—in the United Kingdom, they have been sold only since 2007—and that it is possible that they pose some risk because they contain ingredients other than nicotine. "But it is likely to be very small and substantially smaller than that arising from tobacco smoking," it continued. "With appropriate product standards to minimise exposure to other ingredients, it should be possible to reduce risks to physical health still further."

And then: "The available data suggest that they are unlikely to exceed 5% of those associated with smoked tobacco products, and may well be substantially lower than this figure."

In the report, John Britton, an epidemiologist and professor at the University of Nottingham who chairs the college's Tobacco Advisory Group, said: "This report lays to rest almost all of the concerns over these products, and concludes that, with sensible regulation, electronic cigarettes have the potential to make a major contribution towards preventing the premature death, disease and social inequalities in health that smoking currently causes in the UK."

Another recently published study was the first to look at the long(ish) health effects of e-cigarette use. Scientists from a number of institutions, including the University College London and the Centers for Disease Control and Prevention in the United States, found that, over six months, of the study's 181 British participants, those who had switched completely from combustible cigarettes to e-cigarettes or other nicotine replacement therapies had significantly lower levels of toxic chemicals and cancer-causing substances in their systems than those who were still lighting up.[70]

And yet, ask people on the street about e-cigarettes and heat-not-burn products and a good portion of them will give you either a quizzical "Huh?" or a rolling of the eyes and a tongue-lashing that they're interchangeable with cigarettes and just as dangerous. A 2017 survey by the United Kingdom's Action on Smoking and Health found that only 13 per cent of respondents recognized that e-cigarettes were substantially less harmful than combustible ones, while 26 per cent, up from 8.1 per cent in 2013, believed they were just as harmful as cigarettes, or more so. But a review of the evidence finds that almost all of the 2.9 million adults using such products in Great Britain are current smokers or ex-smokers, most of whom are using the devices to help them quit smoking or to prevent them going back to cigarettes. And less than 1 per cent of them are adults or youth who have never smoked before.[71] To me, that's wonderful news!

Following in the footsteps of their colleagues in the United Kingdom, many health experts are beginning to think differently or, at the very least, keeping their minds more open to the possibility that e-cigarettes and heat-not-burn products may help smokers quit. At the Ontario Institute for Cancer Research in Canada, for example, Dr. Geoffrey Fong, with grants from Canadian and American funding agencies, is gauging the impact of e-cigarette technology and government policies that regulate their sale. "We know how harmful standard combustible cigarettes are to human health. Regular smokers increase their risk of death by 50 per cent and on average they will lose 10 years of their life from smoking," said Fong, the founder and chief principal investigator of the International Tobacco Control Policy Evaluation Project. "E-cigarettes may provide a safer system of nicotine delivery and serve as an aid in quitting smoking, but they may also expose nonsmokers to nicotine consumption, which could lead to tobacco use. Because of this, it is very important that we rigorously evaluate the public health consequences of these products."[72]

In the United States, Mitch Zeller, director of the FDA's Center for Tobacco Products, which is responsible for e-cigarette regulations, has acknowledged that the new products present a formidable challenge to the idea that nicotine is dangerous.

"Electronic cigarettes have become the poster child for the questions that, on a societal level, we need to be asking about nicotine," he told *Rolling Stone* magazine. "How could the same compound associated with so much death and disease be so safe that you can buy it without a doctor's prescription? The answer is that it's about the delivery mechanism, not the drug. None of them have easy answers."[73]

In other words, while nicotine may be addictive, *how* it is delivered into one's body may mean the difference between life and death.

Between *many* lives and deaths.

Even more recently—in the summer of 2017—Scott Gottlieb, commissioner of the FDA, stated that reduced-risk products, in tandem with regulated amounts of nicotine, could help lessen the effect smoking has on health. He said that nicotine, though not benign, is not directly responsible for the tobacco-caused cancer, lung disease, and heart disease that kill hundreds of thousands of Americans each year. Moreover, he continued that the FDA's approach to reducing the devastating toll of tobacco use must be rooted in this foundational understanding: other chemical compounds in tobacco, and in the smoke created by combustion, are primarily to blame for such health harms.[74]

To me, that is an important start.

12

DOING THE UNTHINKABLE

In July 2017, I spent two weeks in Lausanne with PMI executives and scientists, finalizing the board membership and setting priorities for the new Foundation for a Smoke-Free World. The first thing we had to demonstrate was that these products really do lower the death rate. To that end, PMI has submitted an application to the US FDA to market IQOS with a label that states: "This product reduces your risk by [a definite percentage]," that percentage yet to be determined. As I said earlier, studies indicate that the risk of contracting a tobacco-related condition is about 95 per cent less, but without long-term data to support that contention, it's safe to say that the reduced risk is between 80 and 95 per cent—which is good enough for me. The application is exceptionally, mind-bogglingly thorough, including two million pages of research documents—basically all the science PMI has done to date.

During those weeks, I also met with about fifty people—experts, former colleagues, friends who've known me since I started working at WHO—and I was gratified to learn that they were willing to support my decision to work for the foundation because of who I was and what I have done. There were questions, to be sure—big questions and some discomfort. One long-time colleague, Douglas Bettcher, who I had recruited to join WHO almost twenty years earlier, joined me for dinner at an Italian restaurant overlooking Lake Geneva and said: "Derek, you really think this is the way forward? You realize I'm going to have to tell the boss about this?"

I replied: "It's okay. I'm seeing him tomorrow."

The next morning, PMI's director of global policy, who'd come to Connecticut back in May 2015 to make the pitch for me to come to Geneva, drove me to WHO's headquarters. The irony did not escape me: I, the principal architect of the global tobacco control treaty and the most fervent antitobacco activist, bar none, was being driven to the building by a PMI executive in a PMI car.

The director of global policy had to wait outside since tobacco company employees are not permitted on WHO premises—fallout from their years of lies and underhanded lobbying. But in setting up my meetings, I was very clear about what I was doing, and the officials simply kept the information quiet.

The guard on the security desk was the same one who'd been there when I'd worked at WHO. We greeted each other warmly.

I thought, *You don't realize you are breezily welcoming someone who is coming to speak to the bosses about the unthinkable.*

Many people who stopped to say hello in the coffee foyer at the front of the building probably thought I was there because the new director-general, Tedros Adhanom, a politician, academic, and public health authority from Ethiopia, was recruiting me to come back. Of course, he wasn't. I didn't even have a meeting set up with him.

One former colleague took my news in stride and said he would put me in touch with an Ethiopian physician who was trying to stem the damage from combustible cigarettes in his country.

Another former colleague, who I think of as the consummate British public servant, listened as I told him I was not there to negotiate or tell people what they should think or do.

"I just want to inform people what is going to happen," I said. "I don't want them to be blindsided by me leading the foundation."

At one point in the hour-long meeting, he noted: "You do realize this may be the last time you will be welcomed at WHO."

I replied: "The next time I come back, I hope I will be able to convince you to become a grantee of the foundation."

He didn't reply. He just smiled.

No one asked if I was doing it for the money. They knew me too well to think that, and I was very clear about the salary structures. They would be in line with those of other foundations of the same size—that is, a bit more than salaries at academic institutions.

But they were concerned about the separation of church and state, as in PMI and the foundation, especially because the one was financing the other. Would there be continued interference? A blurring or softening of research results if they were not in PMI's favor? And what about lobbying practices? As recently as July 2017, Philip Morris had been the subject of an extensive investigation by the Reuters News Agency. Their findings indicated that PMI was working in clandestine fashion to block or weaken provisions in the very global tobacco control treaty I had helped orchestrate on the grounds of it being a "regulatory runaway train" run by "anti-tobacco extremists."

Called "The Philip Morris Files," the series relied on a cache of e-mails, internal company documents, and interviews with current and former company employees to reveal a secretive "offensive that stretches from the Americas to Africa to Asia, from hardscrabble tobacco fields to the halls of political power, in what may be one of the broadest corporate lobbying efforts in existence."[75]

Tom Snyder, PMI's vice president of communications, responded to Reuters with a statement that noted the company is part of a highly regulated industry, which speaks with governments as part of its everyday business and has a goal to replace cigarettes with less harmful alternatives. "We believe we have something to contribute and we look for a range of legitimate opportunities to express our views to decision-makers," it read. "The fact that Reuters has seen internal emails discussing our engagement with governments does not make those interactions inappropriate. We believe that the active participation of public health experts, policy-makers, scientists, and the industry is the best way to effectively address tobacco regulations in the genuine interest of today's billion smokers."[76]

What, my former colleagues asked, about *that*?

I understood their concerns perfectly. The response to the Reuters series was a masterful piece of spin that didn't say much of anything at all—and really, what could the company say? There still are some dirty marketing tactics out there, and not only by PMI. As I learned at PepsiCo and practically every other big company I have encountered, they can have a team practicing "dark arts" even as they try to make positive changes. It's hard to cut a cancer out willy-nilly. Dangerous, even. Positive change starts at the top and trickles down, and it takes time to get everyone on board. And even if there are still problems, they don't negate good intentions and the billions of dollars poured into research and the transformation of cigarette factories in places such as Bologna, Italy; Aspropy-rgos, Greece; St. Petersburg, Russia; and Dresden, Germany.

"Look at the multi-billion-dollar investment in a research and development facility, with scientists drawn from the cutting edges of the field," I said. "That's a fact. The sheer level and minutiae of systems biology they have developed is far beyond what we have ever known before."

I noted that PMI had agreed to independent assessments of its research results, not only because it was politically expedient but also because its scientists were excited to share their findings and be critiqued by the best of the best. And PMI was committed to working with tobacco farmers to change over their crops as needs for tobacco decline.

As for the fear of interference, I said there needed to be a Chinese firewall between the foundation and PMI—and, in the future, other tobacco companies as they increase their commitment to reduced-risk products.

"There has to be a formula for dialogue, the same kind of model that was there for the development of an AIDS vaccine and malaria treatments," I said. "It's the same principle I've been working with for years: public-private partnerships."

Not that it was a completely smooth road to forging an agreement, I admitted. What agreement ever is? But in the spirit of Brundtland's rule all those years ago during the global antitobacco treaty negotiations that nothing is agreed until everything is agreed, I was ready to walk away from the foundation until such time as PMI made its commitment on paper to the funding. Legal documents, duly signed and notarized, made this endeavor go far beyond a handshake agreement and a feeling of trust!

Throughout the negotiations and my meetings with experts and former colleagues, over the days and weeks and months of discussions and e-mails, I kept thinking of what Harlan Cleveland told a group of us in the late 1990s: the most important life lesson he'd learned was how to live with constructive ambiguity.

That was going to be my life for the foreseeable future.

■

As I walked out of the WHO building, I noticed the bronze statue of a blind man being led out of the forest by his determined son. It is a commemoration of the first-ever public-private partnership between the organization and Merck & Company, Inc. to combat river blindness in Africa.

If PMI came through on its promise to eradicate combustible tobacco products and other companies followed suit, I wondered how the effort would be depicted here. Perhaps one day a bronze statue in the form of a tobacco plant would pay tribute to that accomplishment.

In the interim, before the foundation was officially launched, in an effort to get permission to label heat-not-burn products as "reduced risk," the company submitted millions of pages to the FDA for review.[77] Calantzopoulos has held true to his

promise to place what in the past would have been propri-
etary research in the public domain, available for anybody
to test and replicate. He said as much to a reporter from *Die
Zeit* magazine in Germany, just after the company announced
construction of the new IQOS factory in Dresden. The reporter
wondered why, after Philip Morris's lies to the public for
decades about the risk tobacco posed to unborn children, the
addictive properties of nicotine, and the dangers of secondhand smoke, the company should be believed now.

"Four hundred people work at our research centre in Neuchâtel, most of whom were at pharmaceutical or biochemical
companies before," Calantzopoulos replied. "One of them
comes from the systems biology department at Novartis, for
example. All those people did not come to end their careers
and produce fake science in the future."

The reporter commented that in the past, that is exactly
how things looked.

Said Calantzopoulos: "I'm not asking you to trust me. I'm
asking you to check our data! The aerosol from Heat Sticks can
be quickly analyzed, compared to cigarette smoke. You immediately recognize the reduction in dangerous substances."

In that same interview, Calantzopoulos noted that clinical
studies on patients are proving more difficult for two related
reasons: each individual test can cost up to €40,000, which
means the cost for representative findings will be between
€8 million and €10 million, and who has the means to fund
that right now? Tobacco companies have the means. And one

company is willing to do it right now. Even though PMI is offering to pay to have its data studied and verified by independent institutes, there will always be someone, or some group, that claims the outcome has been bought.

"So, we need an independent body that takes the money and determines how the studies should be run," he continued.[78]

I couldn't agree more. The very fact that PMI submitted its entire data set to the FDA for review is a sign of good faith and—I believe—a sign of even better things to come. This way, experts can reanalyze the data in any fashion they want, with or without bias. The pharmaceutical industry has never done anything like this. In its effort to build the public's trust from the ground up, PMI is setting the scene for a level of transparency that is higher than anything we've ever seen before. It is also setting the stage for a new generation of thinkers to continue what I with my colleagues began over twenty years ago. I think we have done what we can when it comes to taxing tobacco products and banning marketing. Now we need to cultivate thinkers who can build beyond what we have already accomplished. To make the field more exciting. More personal. And more responsive, to both consumers, farmers, and manufacturers.

The bottom line is that, unknown to most people in the public sector, the tobacco industry has been working for years on advances in molecular and cellular biology, DNA research, earlier detections of diseases such as cancer, and more accurate methods with which to measure environmental exposure for nonsmokers. Although much of the work has already been presented at international conferences and published in over two hundred peer review journals, including *The Journal of Cell Biology* and *Nature*, the FDA officials who review the application still have a massive job ahead of them. And of course, there is going to be the question: Can they trust the scientists? No one else is doing this kind of research.

It's time to climb out of the box and into the real world.

■

In September 2017, the Foundation for a Smoke-Free World was incorporated in Delaware with initial funding from PMI of about $80 million annually over the next twelve years—$960 million altogether. If it all works out (remember, constructive ambiguity!), that money will only be the beginning since we expect to receive funding from other sources as well. More importantly, the grant terms, bylaws, and nonprofit status of the foundation prevent representatives from PMI or other tobacco industries from taking part in its governance and having any influence on funding decisions, strategies, or activities.

The foundation's board members come from the worlds of medicine, business, and agriculture. They include Marian Jacobs, the much-lauded South African public health pediatrician and former dean of the medical school at the University of Cape Town, who was perceptive enough to realize I would do well in epidemiology; Dyborn Chibonga, former CEO of the National Smallholder Farmers' Association of Malawi who now works for the Alliance for a Green Revolution in Africa as the regional head for Malawi and Mozambique; Michael Sagner, a pioneer of lifestyle medicine in Europe who serves as president of the European Society of Preventive Medicine; Lisa Gable, an expert on public-private partnerships whose extensive resumé includes serving as president of the Healthy Weight Commitment Foundation that was a key part of former first lady Michelle Obama's "Let's Move!" initiative; and Zoe Feldman, once a consultant and scientist at PepsiCo who is now an entrepreneur with a firm that focuses on seed ventures as well as early-stage and private-equity deals for emerging restaurants and other parts of the hospitality industry. We at the foundation are our own bosses, running an organization with an independent research agenda, ownership of our data, complete freedom to publish, and strict protections against any conflict of interest. With all of our research findings in the public domain, for anyone's easy access, I believe this sets the highest of bars for corporate philanthropy in general: a formula that proves tobacco companies haven't had a role in the research and a peer review process that will help judge the best science and what centers the foundation should support.

Initial activities will focus on four areas: research smoking harm reduction and build research capacity through academic centers of excellence, exploring which interventions can best reduce harm and help smokers to quit, monitor progress around the world on harm-reduction measures, and identify alternative crops and livelihoods for tobacco farmers as the demand for tobacco decreases.

Certainly, there is a long way to go. Changing attitudes, both outside an organization and within, is one of the hardest things I have ever tried to do. I was not surprised when, after the foundation launched its website in mid-September 2017, we received an e-mail from WHO asking for two sections to be edited in order to cut out two facts. First, reference to my being the expert who led development of the world's foremost treaty on tobacco control and was its primary architect. And second, reference to WHO by name in a section on research that states what we do "will complement and add depth to reports already produced by entities such as the World Health Organization and Bloomberg Philanthropies."

As if, in one fell stroke, my contributions, my more than twenty years of hard work, and my leadership on the tobacco control treaty, could become null and void! And as if WHO's research should only be acknowledged by a select group of people and organizations!

Experts in a few countries, such as Australia, which bans the sale of e-cigarettes that contain nicotine, have taken a hard line because they have always been tough on smoking. "We shouldn't treat smokers as guinea pigs," Becky Freeman, a tobacco control expert at Australia's University of Sydney, told *The Guardian* newspaper last summer. "We have no long-term evidence for the safety of e-cigarettes or their efficacy as quit aids. The threshold for whether these products are safe is always about how they fare in comparison to cigarettes. But I can't think of anything more harmful to human health than cigarettes, so that's a pretty low bar."[79]

True to form, Stanton Glantz of the University of California, San Francisco, in a blog post, likened the foundation's independence to that of "all past industry front groups," conceivably in which we purport to support one agenda while clandestinely serving another, more nefarious one.[80] And I wasn't surprised when WHO's official response to the creation of the foundation was a resounding rejection because PMI is funding it, even while engaged in large-scale lobbying and expensive litigation against evidence-based tobacco control policies. In a news release, the organization acknowledged there are many unanswered questions about tobacco harm reduction but it stressed that the research needed to answer these questions should not be funded by tobacco companies because of their propensity to mislead and obfuscate. "This includes promoting so-called light and mild tobacco products as an alternative to quitting, while being fully aware that those products were not less harmful to health," the release stated. "Such misleading conduct continues today with companies, including PMI, marketing tobacco products in ways that misleadingly suggest that some tobacco products are less harmful than others."[81]

I have gently pointed out that the foundation is not PMI, nor interchangeable with PMI. That it is an independent entity devoted to ending the deadly toll caused by combustible smoking around the world. And that it welcomes funding from elsewhere: we are actively seeking partnerships that will help the foundation achieve its stated goals.

Accepting this requires a new mindset. To that end, I've already been working with the International Actuarial Association, which rates the risk of various activities to create templates used by health and life insurance companies. As a result of their assessment, e-cigarettes will be treated as less dangerous than combustible ones. It's a small but important step forward.

■

I know that I've jumped into a much bigger fire than PepsiCo ever was, if only because I built my reputation on fighting the tobacco industry and being an antitobacco rock star. Sometimes, it feels like a conflagration. But I haven't changed. I'm still doing what I have always done, driven by the same pressing desire to prevent disease and improve public health in the most effective way I see possible. From where I stand, preventing sixty million deaths over the next twenty years sounds wonderful.

Yes, I am now with a foundation that is funded by PMI, but I am not beholden to that company's history or whatever dark marketing arts it may still practice today. I have my independence, my wealth of experience, and the conviction that, until we discover a better way to get people to easily quit smoking, this is the most effective way to stem its terrible toll. And we at the foundation do not want to work alone. Instead, we want to partner with governments, with NGOs, and, if possible, with other tobacco companies on smoking-cessation campaigns and on products that really do reduce risk. That is both the company's and the foundation's great challenge. It's scary. It's exciting. And for me, it's a near blank slate on which I can inscribe the experience from a lifetime of working in the field.

Throughout it all, I've partnered with and been inspired by courageous, visionary people. By Hannes Botha at the South African Medical Research Council, Gro Harlem Brundtland at WHO, and Kelly Brownell at Yale; by "Inspirer-in-Chief" Bill Clinton at the Clinton Global Initiative, Indra Nooyi at PepsiCo, and Adrian Gore at Vitality. Now, I count André Calantzopoulos of PMI among them, for he has become an invaluable ally in the battle against combustible cigarettes.

If that's unthinkable, so be it.

AFTERWORD

On a sunny weekend in September 2017, just before the public learned of my full-time move to the Foundation for a Smoke-Free World, I sat in my study in Southport, writing a two-thousand-word essay on why I was doing so for *The Lancet*, one of the world's oldest and best-known medical journals. I have known its editor-in-chief, Richard Horton, for over twenty years, and there is no medical journalist I respect more. He is one of the stalwarts when it comes to being cautious about tobacco company claims, but he is also willing to listen to other points of view.

I had arranged a phone call with him the week before to break the news. My only regret is that I couldn't see the expression of shock—and perhaps horror—on his face.

"Oh my God," he said from his office in London. "Oh my God. Oh my God."

He was concerned for me, to say the least. But he also had the presence of mind to know he had trusted my judgment in the public health arena in the past, so he wanted to hear more about my vision for the future. He asked me to write a piece to describe what the foundation could do, address the issue of the independence, and talk about what has happened in the past as a way of responding to the criticism that would inevitably fall upon my head.

How could I distill history into two thousand words? *My* history? The scholarly papers and letters I've written for *The Lancet* itself go back a quarter century, in effect following my trajectory through successive jobs and responsibilities. The first was a paper in 1993 about South Africa's health service. In 2003, I wrote a letter taking issue with a paper that contained suggestions that the proposed draft text for WHO's Framework Convention on Tobacco Control was "feeble" and "meaningless."

"There are some misconceptions about what a framework convention is and what makes it effective," I wrote. "A framework convention is what the name signifies: a framework. Within this framework, protocols will be negotiated on specific subjects, with detailed, binding provisions on all important issues set out."

With regard to issues such as advertising, promotion, and sponsorship of tobacco products, I stated that the language in the draft text makes it clear that the ultimate objective is a complete advertising ban and provides for such a ban through binding declarations in accordance with WHO and World Bank policy. "Earlier negotiations have witnessed polarised debates about the political and constitutional limitations on complete bans of advertising, promotion, and sponsorship," I continued. "The fact that few countries have enacted a complete ban illustrates the difficulty of implementing such legislation domestically, especially on a universal level. A framework convention cannot go further than the political will of the negotiators at a given time."[82]

Years later, when I was at Vitality, I wrote a paper that was published in January 2014—a retrospective piece on the treaty by one who had been in the thick of things. I noted then that the treaty's many references to tobacco product design and regulation failed to anticipate alternative nicotine-de-livery products that did not contain tobacco even though, in the view of many experts, the products have the potential to disrupt many traditional aspects of tobacco control. Such developments meant that WHO should revisit its policies on nicotine versus tobacco, I said, invoking a comment Brundt-land made more than ten years earlier.

"Despite our concerns about these clear differences in position, we are committed to hearing how the tobacco com-panies do propose to reduce the harm that their products cause," she said during public hearings for the treaty in 2000. "Our Scientific Advisory Committee is charged with propos-ing appropriate national and international tobacco product regulatory frameworks. We have invited tobacco company scientists to provide their views on product modification to this Committee."[83]

And now, on this sunny weekend, here I was, not a tobacco company scientist, to be sure—but one who was trying to bridge the gap between the two sides.

Because I believe in the science.

Because I believe that with the right kind of leadership, companies can change.

Because saving lives is paramount.

I began to write. "I believe this is the time to raise our ambition for what is possible and desirable in tobacco control."

And: "What drives me to action and to accept this challenge is the massive, unprecedented potential to join a global effort to accelerate the decline in tobacco deaths and to prove wrong those who still project a billion smoking-related deaths this century."

There have been some heartening developments. In October 2017, I spoke in Washington, DC, at the annual conference of the Food and Drug Law Institute. I was fortunate that my speech followed that of Mitch Zeller, director of the FDA's Center for Tobacco Products. I consider him a true intellectual leader in the world of tobacco control, with a mind open to tackling a long-term, deadly problem. He focused on the challenges of reducing the risks associated with smoking, helping smokers to quit, and ensuring that kids aren't able to start.

"You all have an equal shot to take part in rule making," he said.

I agreed, telling the audience that I assume "all" refers to anyone with a material interest and with knowledge and insights to contribute to tobacco control. This includes academics, scientists from the industries working on ways to reduce risk and improve cessation, lead government regulators, NGOs, users of tobacco and related products—and the Foundation for a Smoke-Free World. And what we need to recognize is the major shift going on right now in how we tackle the problem of smoking: from attempting to eradicate it altogether toward focusing more on regulation of nicotine and how it is delivered.

I said we all share a common goal in accelerating the end of smoking among the one billion smokers in the world, and that the foundation is part of a new movement that is disrupting the status quo. And it is only to be expected that people get upset every time such a disruption occurs—like the Luddites of the nineteenth century, and those who protest genetically modified crops or driverless cars. Invariably, the first response involves fear and urgent calls for censure or an outright ban. Yet, even as these calls are made, the early acolytes of these new movements are able to find benefits and organize others to benefit, too. Remember when former US president Ronald Reagan assured doubters about his decision to meet with former Soviet president Mikhail Gorbachev about ending the Cold War? He said, "We trust, but verify."

I told the audience that very principle drives the foundation. We will make our case not by asking people to trust us, but through independent oversight, transparency, and public reporting. This is about defining a way to achieve a goal and verifying whether or not we're doing it. That means people should study our plans, read our mission statement, and let us know what else we can do to provide the needed verification of independence.

Don't censor, I concluded. Communicate. Be skeptical, sure, but participate in a dialogue about stemming the deadly toll that smoking takes, and will continue to take in the future. Because that is what this new movement is about.

I think—I hope—I was received well.

Elsewhere, positive responses to the foundation and its mission have come from the worlds of health, ethics, medicine, and agriculture, all of which want more innovation in the field of harm reduction and know that such innovations cost lots of money. Applications for grants have exceeded my expectations, both in terms of number and quality. The applicants include cutting-edge scientists and far-seeing entrepreneurs from major universities and centers in places as diverse as Boston and Bangalore, Italy and Peru.

In December 2017, Richard Smith, former editor of the *BMJ*, who has known me for a quarter century, wrote a blog calling me the leading strategic thinker in the global battle against noncommunicable diseases, be it at WHO, PepsiCo, and now—despite the confounding nature of my decision—maybe even at the Foundation for a Smoke-Free World.

> *There is a logic to Yach's move … The appearance of e-cigarettes is changing the world of tobacco as railways changed canals and digital images changed film. How should tobacco companies react? If they react wrongly they may follow Kodak, who failed to respond correctly to the appearance of digital images, into oblivion. Philip Morris International seems to have bet that e-cigarettes will be the future, and so there is business logic to funding a Foundation for a Smoke-Free World … Nobody will benefit from creating further division among public health people and organisations. People, I believe, should not only be talking to the tobacco industry, but to each other with mutual respect.*[84]

Hoorah!

I am also gratified and humbled that the foundation has been featured in an ethics course at Harvard T.H. Chan School of Public Health, having been added to the list of suggested topics for students' term projects in the course called Social and Individual Responsibility for Health. The gist of it is thus: Harvard researchers are forbidden from accepting money from tobacco companies because of their outright lies, obfuscations, and underhanded lobbying. But with PMI's announcement that it is striving for a world free of smoking and will transfer about $1 billion over an extended period to an independent, nonprofit foundation—namely, us—which offers grants for research on limiting tobacco-related harm, the faculty needs ethical advice on whether the school should engage with the foundation and, if so, on what terms. The reading list includes the piece I wrote for *The Lancet* on why I agreed to create and run the foundation and a book by Harvard law professor Robert Mnookin, *Bargaining with the Devil: When to Negotiate, When to Fight*, which contains practical advice for dealing with someone, or something, you don't trust and even fear may do you harm.[85]

I welcome that kind of approach because I welcome debate. All I'm asking is that antitobacco activists, former colleagues, governments, universities, and organizations such as WHO keep an open mind and consider all sides rather than hastily jumping to ill-informed, knee-jerk conclusions. Given the dark history of tobacco companies, I know it is a lot to ask. But I went through those very same mental contortions when I was considering taking the job, and I realized that the risk was worth it.

In the end—or, better, my new beginning—I am left with an overwhelming sense of responsibility to the issue, to my colleagues and teachers who have always had faith in me and my decisions, and to my family. To my sister, Dianna, who runs our family foundation, chairs the board at the University of Cape Town, and has used Nicorette Gum for more than thirty years. To my brother, Theodore, a property developer in Cape Town who long ago eclipsed me in swimming feats, and to my youngest brother, Jonathan, who lives in Bangalore and develops malls in India. To my wife, Yasmin, my stalwart support and sounding board, and my son, Julian, who was there when the global tobacco treaty was signed.

Most of all, to my parents. To my mother, who through a Herculean effort of will, somehow managed to cut down her smoking when her grandchildren were born. And to my late father, whose gentle, insistent words I still hear every day.

Be brave. Be tough. Take risks, don't give up and, most of all, don't be afraid to fail.

ACKNOWLEDGMENTS

Writing this book has allowed me to revisit and explore the momentous forces that have shaped who I am today. Three come immediately to mind: growing up in apartheid South Africa, the historic 1978 Alma-Ata conference that identified primary health care as the key to attaining "Health for All," and the lawsuits against the U.S. tobacco industry in the 1990s that brought to light its shady tactics and shameless lies.

But even more forceful are the people I've encountered over the years—people who have played key roles in shaping my ideas and helped me to make sometimes unexpected life decisions. They are family members, close friends, academic mentors who somehow seemed to know me better than I knew myself, and professional colleagues who have both supported me and called me out when they thought I was wrong. If only I could name you all!

Of course, I do need to highlight some names. My wife and life partner, Yasmin von Schirnding, has been with me for over 40 years, my biggest cheerleader and most incisive critic. No matter if it's a conversation about health issues, scientific advances, or career direction, it is you I want to speak to first thing in the morning and last thing at night.

Others I must mention: Marian Jacobs, Hannes Botha, Debbie Bradshaw, Gro Harlem Brundtland, Indra Nooyi, Adrian Gore, and the late George Comstock. All of you played powerful roles in shaping what positions I would have, where I would focus my energies, and what really mattered in the pursuit of health for all.

Throughout my career, I've been lucky to work with brilliant young people who have constantly challenged the status quo, suggested areas of research I had never considered, and helped pave the way for me to refresh old ideas and explore new possibilities. Heather Wipfli, Gillian Christie, Elle Alexander are three of the most exceptional minds in this exceptional group.

Finally, I have learned that it is easy to think about a book and even map out its content in depth, but it takes a lot more discipline, writing ability, and attention to detail to actually get it done. For that, I am so grateful to Lisa Fitterman for helping turn ideas and long stories into tight, compelling chapters that follow my life's arc, and to Sarah Scott, my publisher, for holding my hand throughout a long period of gestation and work. All errors are, of course, mine!

ENDNOTES

1   *World Health Statistics 2017: Monitoring Health for the SDGs (Sustainable Development Goals)*, http://apps.who.int/iris/bitstream/10665/255336/1/9789241565486-eng.pdf?ua=1 (accessed July 15, 2017).

2   *WHO Report on the Global Tobacco Epidemic 2017*, www.who.int/tobacco/global_report/2017/en/ (accessed May 5, 2017).

3   Declaration of Alma-Ata International Conference on Primary Health Care, Alma-Ata, USSR, 6–12 September 1978, www.who.int/publications/almaata_declaration_en.pdf (accessed May 6, 2017).

4   D. Yach, "The Impact of Political Violence on Health and Health Services in Cape Town, South Africa, 1986: Methodological Problems and Preliminary Results," *American Journal of Public Health* 78, no. 7 (July 1988):772–8, http://ajph.aphapublications.org/doi/pdf/10.2105/AJPH.78.7.772 (accessed June 15, 2017).

5   D. Yach, "Economic Aspects of Smoking in South Africa," *South African Medical Journal* 62, no. 6 (July 31, 1982):167–70.

6   *South African Medical Journal* 73, no. 7 (April 2, 1988).

7   A.J. Brink, "The Smoking Trail: Research Shows a Path of Death and Destruction," *South African Medical Journal* 73, no. 7 (April 2, 1988):385–87.

8   Mia Malan and Rosemary Leaver, "Political Change in South Africa: New Tobacco Control and Public Health Policies," World Bank Group, October 2011, 126, in *Tobacco Control Policy: Strategies, Successes, and Setbacks*, co-publication of World Bank and Research for International Tobacco (RITC), Joy De Beyer and Linda Waverly, http://siteresources.worldbank.org/INTETC/Resources/ 375990-1113921158191/2850-Ch06.pdf (accessed June 6, 2017).

9   Mia Malan and Rosemary Leaver, "Political Change in South Africa: New Tobacco Control and Public Health Policies," 127, in *Tobacco Control Policy: Strategies, Successes, and Setbacks*, co-publication of World Bank and Research for International Tobacco (RITC), Joy De Beyer and Linda Waverly, http://siteresources.worldbank.org/INTETC/ Resources/375990-1113921158191/2850-Ch06.pdf (accessed June 6, 2017).

10 "Tobacco Growers Stand By for Some Fuming," *The Farmer* (November 4, 1993): photocopy.

11 British American Tobacco Limited, Facsimile to Publics Managers Africa, cc H. Thomson, from Shabanji Opukah, June 6, 1995.

12 British American Tobacco Company Limited, Facsimile to Hilary Thomson, UTC Holdings, from Shabanji Opukah, June 27, 1995.

13 Fernando S. Antezana, Claire M. Chollat-Traquet, and Derek Yach, "Health for All in the 21st Century," produced for WHO, 1998, www.who.int/iris/handle/10665/55721 (accessed July 5, 2017).

14 "The Growing Danger of Non-Communicable Diseases: Acting Now to Reverse Course," World Bank Human Development Network, September 2011.

15 Allyn Lise Taylor, "Making the World Health Organization Work: A Legal Framework for Universal Access to the Conditions for Health," *American Journal of Law and Medicine* 18 (1992):301–47.

16 Ruth Roemer, *Legislative Action to Combat the World Tobacco Epidemic* (Geneva: World Health Organization, 1993).

17 Lakshmi Chaudhry, "Chitra Subramanian and Bofors: The Myth of the Lone Crusader," *Firstpost* (online), www.firstpost.com/india/chitra-subramaniam-and-bofors-the-myth-of-the-lone-crusader-289498.html (accessed July 16, 2017).

18 Gro Harlem Brundtland, International Speech to the 51st World Health Assembly, May 13, 1988, www.malaria.org/SPEECH.HTM (accessed June 30, 2017).

19 World Health Organization, Director-General/Former Director-General Dr. Gro Harlem Brundtland, www.who.int/dg/brundtland/en/ (accessed June 30, 2017).

20 "New broom at WHO," BBC News, July 21, 1998, http://news.bbc.co.uk/2/hi/136702.stm (accessed June 28, 2017).

21 Dr. Gro Harlem Brundtland, Director-General Elect, the World Health Organization, Speech to the 51st World Health Assembly, Geneva, May 13 1988, http://www.malaria.org/SPEECH.HTM (accessed July 5, 2017).

22 *1999 Annual Report from WHO's Tobacco Free Initiative*, http://forces-nl.org/WHO/pdf/annualtf.pdf (accessed July 5, 2017).

23 "Channel the Outrage Project," WHO Tobacco Free Initiative, www.who.int/tobacco/research/ngo/en/ (accessed July 5, 2017).

24 Philip Morris, "New WHO Director-General Makes International Regulation of Tobacco One of the WHO's Central Objectives: A Report on the 51st World Health Assembly and 102nd Meeting of the WHO's Executive Board," (2065285220), http://legacy.library.ucsf.edu/tid/spt83c00/pdf?search=%222065285220%22, 1998 (accessed July 6, 2017).

25 Report of the Committee of Experts on Tobacco Industry Documents, "Tobacco Company Strategies to Undermine Tobacco Control Activities at the World Health Organization," July 2000, www.who.int/tobacco/en/who_inquiry.pdf?ua=1 (accessed July 6, 2017).

26 C.J.L. Murray and A.D. Lopez, eds., "The Global Burden of Disease: A Comprehensive Assessment of Mortality and Disability from Diseases, Injuries and Risk Factors in 1990, and Projected to 2020," Harvard School of Public Health on behalf of the World Health Organization and the World Bank, 1996, http://apps.who.int/iris/bitstream/10665/41864/1/0965546608_eng.pdf (accessed July 2, 2017).

27 Video Q&A: "Tobacco-related Mortality: Past, Present and Future. An interview with Alan Lopez," *BMC Medicine* (October 21, 2014), video, https://bmcmedicine.biomedcentral.com/articles/10.1186/s12916-014-0162-x (accessed July 5, 2017).

28 Laksmi Chaudhry, "Chitra Subramanian and Bofors: The Myth of the Lone Crusader," *Firstpost* (online), April 26, 2012, www.firstpost.com/india/chitra-subramaniam-and-bofors-the-myth-of-the-lone-crusader-289498.html (accessed July 17, 2017).

29 Note from Simon Millson to Martin Broughton, "World Economic Forum, Security Society or Sterile Society? Preserving Freedom of Choice while Protecting Public Health," speech and background briefing, January 27, 1999.

30 "WHO Framework Convention on Tobacco Control," May 21, 2003, United Nations Treaty Collection, https://treaties.un.org/pages/ViewDetails.aspx?src=TREATY&mtdsg_no=IX-4&chapter=9&lang=en (accessed May 1, 2017).

31 Derek Yach, Corinna Hawkes, Joanne E. Epping-Jordan, and Sarah Galbraith, "The World Health Organization's Framework Convention on Tobacco Control: Implications for Global Epidemics of Food-related Deaths and Disease," *Journal of Public Health Policy* 24: 3/4 (2003): 274–90, www.researchgate.net/profile/Derek_Yach/publication/5390684_The_World_Health_Organization%27s_Framework_Convention_on_Tobacco_Control_Implications_for_Global_Epidemics_of_Food-Related_Deaths_and_Disease/links/54d4f4330cf2970e4e63f749.pdf (accessed May 5, 2017).

32 World Health Organization, "Global Strategy on Diet, Physical Activity and Health," www.who.int/dietphysicalactivity/strategy/ eb11344/strategy_english_web.pdf (accessed May 5, 2017).

33 Sarah Bosely, "Sugar Industry Threatens to Scupper WHO," *The Guardian*, April 21, 2003, www.theguardian.com/society/2003/ apr/21/usnews.food (accessed July 14, 2017).

34 Health and Medicine Division, U.S. National Academies of Science, Engineering and Medicine, "Dietary Reference Intakes for Energy, Carbohydrate, Fiber, Fat, Fatty Acids, Cholesterol, Protein, and Amino Acids," September 5, 2002, www.nationalacademies.org/hmd/ Reports/2002/Dietary-Reference-Intakes-for-Energy-Carbohydrate-Fiber-Fat-Fatty-Acids-Cholesterol-Protein-and-Amino-Acids.aspx (accessed May 15, 2017).

35 William R. Steiger, Special Assistant to the Secretary for International Affairs, to the Honorable J.W. Lee, MD, Director-General of the World Health Organization, letter, January 5, 2004, https://cspinet.org/ sites/default/files/attachment/steigerltr.pdf (accessed June 6, 2017).

36 Derek Yach and Corinna Hawkes, "Towards a WHO Long-term Strategy for Prevention and Control of Leading Chronic Diseases," World Health Organization, May 2004, 5, www.who.int/chp/knowledge/ publications/en/LONG%20TERM%20STRATEGY%20Yach.pdf (accessed May 6, 2017).

37 Derek Yach and Corinna Hawkes, "Towards a WHO Long-term Strategy for Prevention and Control of Leading Chronic Diseases," World Health Organization, May 2004, www.who.int/chp/knowledge/ publications/en/LONG%20TERM%20STRATEGY%20Yach.pdf (accessed May 6, 2017).

38 Derek Yach, Corinna Hawkes, C. Linn Gould, and Karen J. Hofman, "The Global Burden of Chronic Diseases: Overcoming Impediments to Prevention and Control," *Journal of the American Medical Association* 291, no. 21 (2004):2616–22, http://jamanetwork.com/journals/jama/ article-abstract/198852 (accessed May 6, 2017).

39 "Merck Offers Free Distribution of New River Blindness Drug,"
    The New York Times, October 22, 1987, 14, www.nytimes.com/1987/
    10/22/world/merck-offers-free-distribution-of-new-river-blindness-
    drug.html (accessed September 15, 2017).

40 Kelly D. Brownell and Marion Nestle, "The Sweet and Lowdown on
    Sugar," *The New York Times*, January 23, 2004, www.nytimes.com/
    2004/01/23/opinion/the-sweet-and-lowdown-on-sugar.html
    (accessed July 6, 2017).

41 Dan Charles, "How One Man Tried to Slim Down Big Soda From the
    Inside," profile of Derek Yach on *Morning Edition*, National Public
    Radio, January 28, 2013, www.npr.org/sections/thesalt/2013/01/
    28/169733003/how-one-man-tried-to-slim-down-big-soda-from-the-
    inside, 3:40–3:47 (accessed July 9, 2017).

42 Ricardo Uauy, Advisory Opinion Letter as part of application to U.S.
    Citizenship & Immigration Services for O-1 Alien of Extraordinary
    Ability in Sciences Petition by Pepsico, Inc. for Derek Yach, December
    22, 2006, 6.

43 Ricardo Uauy, "Invited Commentary to Yach Editorial," *Public Health
    Nutrition* 11, no. 2 (February 1, 2008):111–12, file:///C:/Users/Lisa/
    AppData/Local/Microsoft/Windows/INetCache/Content.Outlook/
    HQWT27YA/UAUY%20on%20Yach%20(002).pdf (accessed July 27,
    2017).

44 Kaare R. Norum, "Invited Commentary to Yach Editorial: PepsiCo
    Recruitment Strategy Challenged," *Public Health Nutrition* 11, no. 2
    (February 1, 2008):112–13, file:///C:/Users/Lisa/AppData/Local/
    Packages/Microsoft.MicrosoftEdge_8wekyb3d8bbwe/TempState/
    Downloads/kaare20on20yach20editorial.pdf (accessed July 27, 2017).

45 Derek Yach, "Invited Editorial, A Personal View: Food Companies
    and Nutrition for Better Health," *Public Health Nutrition* 11, no. 2
    (February 1, 2008):109–11, file:///C:/Users/Lisa/AppData/Local/
    Microsoft/Windows/INetCache/Content.Outlook/HQWT27YA/
    Derek%20Yach%20Articlephn%20(1).pdf (accessed July 27, 2017).

46   Indra Nooyi, Keynote address at the Food Marketing Institute, Mid-winter conference, Scottsdale, Arizona, January 14, 2008, file:///C:/Users/Lisa/AppData/Local/Microsoft/Windows/ INetCache/Content.Outlook/HQWT27YA/Nooyi%20-%20FMI%20 Speech%20-%20post%20speech%20FINAL%20(1-15-08)%20w%20 logo.pdf (accessed July 27, 2017).

47   Derek Yach, personal notes for a keynote address, Business and Society Conference: "Trading Off: Impactful Business Strategy in Uncertain Times," Tuck School of Business at Dartmouth, February 9, 2012.

48   Marion Nestle, "Pepsi's Answer to Eat Natural: Snackify Beverages and Drinkify Snack," Food Politics blog entry, January 5, 2011, www. foodpolitics.com/?s=fruit+puree+Pepsi (accessed April 20, 2018).

49   Derek Yach, personal notes for a keynote address, Business and Society Conference: "Trading Off: Impactful Business Strategy in Uncertain Times," Tuck School of Business at Dartmouth, February 9, 2012.

50   Michael E. Porter, Mark R. Kramer, and Aldo Sesia, "Discovery Limited: Case Study," *Harvard Business Review* 715-423 (December 4, 2014).

51   Irving Fisher and Eugene Lyman Fisk, *How to Live: Rules for Healthful Living Based on Modern Science* (New York and London: Funk and Wagnalls Company, 1916).

52   Chris Calitz, Keshia M. Pollack, Chris Millard, and Derek Yach, "National Institutes for Health Funding for Behavioral Interventions to Prevent Chronic Diseases," *American Journal of Preventive Medicine* 48, no. 4 (April 2015):462–71, www.ajpmonline.org/article/S0749-3797(14)00620-5/fulltext (accessed August 30, 2017).

53   thevitalityinstitute.org/commission/ (accessed June 5, 2017).

54   "Investing in Prevention: A National Imperative, Key Findings and Recommendations of the Vitality Institute Commission on Health Promotion and the Prevention of Chronic Disease in Working-Age Americans," June 2014, http://thevitalityinstitute.org/site/wp-content/

uploads/2014/06/Vitality_Recommendations2014.pdf (accessed September 7, 2017).

55 "Wir fragen nicht nach Sex" ("We do not ask about sex"), *Der Spiegel* 50 (2014), http://m.spiegel.de/spiegel/print/d-130754227.html (accessed August 30, 2017).

56 Roland Sturm, Ruopeng An, Darren Segal, and Deepak Patel, "A Cash-Back Rebate Program for Healthy Food Purchases in South Africa: Results from Scanner Data," *American Journal of Preventive Medicine* 44, no. 6 (June 2015):567–72, www.ncbi.nlm.nih.gov/pmc/articles/PMC3659342/ (accessed September 7, 2017).

57 Chris Calitz, Keshia M. Pollack, Chris Milliard, and Derek Yach, "National Institutes of Health Funding for Behavioral Interventions to Prevent Chronic Diseases," *American Journal of Preventive Medicine* 48, no. 4 (April 2015):462–71, www.ajpmonline.org/article/S0749-3797(14)00620-5/fulltext (accessed August 30, 2017).

58 Allen Carr, *Easy Way to Stop Smoking* (London: Arcturus Publishing, May 16, 1985).

59 Oxford Journals: *Nicotine & Tobacco Research* 11, no. 10 (October 2009):1175–81, www.ncbi.nlm.nih.gov/pmc/articles/PMC2746836/ (accessed August 11, 2017).

60 Paolo Boffetta, Stephen Hecht, Nigel Gray, Prakash Gupta, and Kurt Straif, "Smokeless Tobacco and Cancer," *The Lancet Oncology* 9, no. 7 (July 2008):667–75, www.thelancet.com/pdfs/journals/lanonc/PIIS1470-2045(08)70173-6.pdf (accessed July 17, 2017).

61 European Commission, Health & Consumer Protection Directorate-General, Scientific Committee on Emerging and Newly Identified Health Risks (SCENIHR), "Health Effects of Smokeless Tobacco Products," 2008, http://ec.europa.eu/health/ph_risk/committees/04_scenihr/docs/scenihr_o_013.pdf (accessed August 5, 2017).

62 Helena Diggard, Graham Errington, Audrey Richter, and Kevin McAdam, "Patterns and Behaviours of Snus Consumption in Sweden," Oxford Journals: *Nicotine & Tobacco Research* 11, no. 10

(October 2009):1175–81, www.ncbi.nlm.nih.gov/pmc/articles/
PMC2746836/ (accessed August 11, 2017).

63 Eurostat—Statistics Explained, "Mortality and Life Expectancy Statistics," June 2017, http://ec.europa.eu/eurostat/statistics-explained/
index.php/Mortality_and_life_expectancy_statistics (accessed August
11, 2017).

64 Derek Yach, "E-cigarettes Save Lives," *The Spectator*, February
21, 2015, www.spectator.co.uk/2015/02/e-cigarettes-save-lives/
(accessed June 6, 2017).

65 André Calantzopoulos, in an interview with BBC Radio 4 program
presenter Dominic O'Connell on November 30, 2016, www.bbc.
co.uk/programmes/p04jhnsw (accessed September 4, 2017).

66 Philip Morris International home page, "Designing a Smoke-Free
Future," www.pmi.com/ (accessed September 15, 2017).

67 A. McNeill, H.S. Brose, R. Calder, S.C. Hitchman, P. Hajek, and
H. McRobbie, "E-cigarettes: An Evidence Update," Public Health
England, August 2015, www.gov.uk/government/uploads/system/
uploads/attachment_data/file/457102/Ecigarettes_an_evidence_
update_A_report_commissioned_by_Public_Health_England_
FINAL.pdf (accessed August 5, 2017).

68 Adrian Gore, Peter Harmer, Marc W. Pfitzer, and Nina Jais, "Can
Insurance Companies Incentivize Their Customers to Be Healthier?,"
Harvard Business Review (June 23, 2017), https://hbr.org/2017/06/
can-insurance-companies-incentivize-their-customers-to-be-healthier
(accessed June 15, 2017).

69 Royal College of Physicians, "Nicotine without Smoke: Tobacco Harm
Reduction. A Report by the Tobacco Advisory Group of the Royal
College of Physicians," April 2016, www.rcplondon.ac.uk/sites/
default/files/media/Documents/Nicotine%20without%20smoke.pdf
(accessed August 5, 2017).

70 Lion Shahab, Maciej L. Goniewicz, Benjamin C. Blount, Jamie
Brown, Ann McNeill, K. Udeni Alwis, June Feng, Lanqing Wang,
and Robert West, "Nicotine, Carcinogen and Toxin Exposure in

Long-Term E-Cigarette and Nicotine Replacement Therapy Users: A Cross-sectional Study," *Annals of Internal Medicine* 166, no. 6 (March 21, 2017):390–400, http://annals.org/aim/article/2599869/nicotine-carcinogen-toxin-exposure-long-term-e-cigarette-nicotine-replacement (accessed August 12, 2017).

71 Action on Smoking and Health (ASH) Fact Sheet, "Use of E-cigarettes (Vapourisers) among Adults in Great Britain," May 2017, file:///C:/Users/Lisa/Downloads/Use-of-e-cigarettes-vapourisers-among-adults-in-Great-Britain-May-2017-2.pdf (accessed September 7, 2017).

72 Ontario Institute for Cancer Research, "OICR's Geoff Fong Receives Major Funding to Examine E-cigarettes and the Impact of Public Health Policy," *OICR News*, August 11, 2016, https://news.oicr.on.ca/2016/08/oicrs-geoff-fong-receives-major-funding-to-examine-e-cigarettes-and-the-impact-of-public-health-policy/ (accessed September 6, 2017).

73 David Amsden, "E-Cigs' Inconvenient Truth: It's Much Safer to Vape," *Rolling Stone* (December 21, 2015), www.rollingstone.com/politics/news/e-cigs-inconvenient-truth-its-much-safer-to-vape-20151221 (accessed September 14, 2017).

74 S. Gottlieb and M. Zelle, "A Nicotine-focused Framework for Public Health," *New England Journal of Medicine* 377 (2017):1111–14.

75 Reuters Investigates, "The Philip Morris Files: The Secrets of the World's Biggest Tobacco Company," July 13, 2017, www.reuters.com/investigates/section/pmi/ (accessed September 20, 2017).

76 Aditya Kalra, Paritosh Bansal, Duff Wilson, and Tom Lasseter, "Treaty Blitz: Inside Philip Morris' Campaign to Subvert the Global Anti-smoking Treaty," Part 1 of Reuters Investigates, "The Philip Morris Files," July 13, 2017, www.reuters.com/investigates/special-report/pmi-who-fctc/ (accessed September 20, 2017).

77 Philip Morris Products S.A. Modified Risk Tobacco Product (MRTP) Applications, www.fda.gov/TobaccoProducts/Labeling/MarketingandAdvertising/ucm546281.htm (accessed September 20, 2017).

78 Marcus Rohwetter, "Wir brauchen etwas mehr Freiheit. André Calant-
    zopoulos, Vorstandschef des Zigarettenriesen Philip Morris Interna-
    tional, plädiert im Interview für das Ende der Zigarette," *Die Zeit*,
    June 21, 2017, www.zeit.de/2017/26/philip-morris-zigaretten-andre-
    calantzopoulos-interview (accessed September 20, 2017).

79 Melissa Davey, "Smoke and Mirrors? Experts Divide over Australia's
    E-cigarettes Ban," *The Guardian* (international edition), August 27,
    2017, www.theguardian.com/society/2017/aug/28/smoke-and-
    mirrors-experts-divide-over-australias-e-cigarettes-ban (accessed
    September 21, 2017).

80 Stanton A. Glantz, "Derek Yach's Journey to the Dark Side Is Now
    Complete," UCSF Center for Tobacco Control, Research and Edu-
    cation faculty blog, September 12, 2017, https://tobacco.ucsf.edu/
    derek-yach%E2%80%99s-journey-dark-side-now-complete (accessed
    September 21, 2017).

81 "WHO Statement on Philip Morris-funded Foundation for a Smoke-
    Free World," September 28, 2017, www.who.int/mediacentre/news/
    statements/2017/philip-morris-foundation/en/ (accessed September
    29, 2017).

82 Derek Yach, "Foundation for a Smoke-Free World," *The Lancet* 390,
    no. 10104 (October 14, 2017):1807–10, www.thelancet.com/journals/
    lancet/article/PIIS0140-6736(17)32602-8/fulltext (accessed October
    14, 2017).

83 WHO. Director-general's response to the tobacco hearings. Octo-
    ber 13, 2000, www.who.int/tobacco/framework/public_hearings/
    dghearings_en.pdf (accessed September 28, 2017).

84 Richard Smith, "A Public Health Witch Hunt—Bad for Everybody,"
    December 19, 2017, http://blogs.bmj.com/bmj/2017/12/19/
    richard-smith-a-public-health-witch-hunt-bad-for-everybody/
    (accessed December 21, 2017).

85 Robert Mnookin, *Bargaining with the Devil: When to Negotiate, When to
    Fight* (New York: Simon and Schuster, 2011).

INDEX

ABOUT
THE
AUTHOR

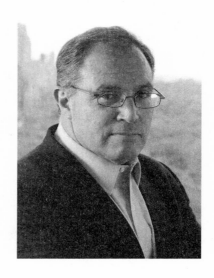

Dr. Derek Yach led the development of the World Health Organization's Framework Convention on Tobacco Control, which imposed strict controls on tobacco throughout the world. After moving to the United States, Yach led the global health effort at the Rockefeller Foundation, and worked as a professor of global health at Yale University. Then he joined PepsiCo, where he worked with the CEO to try to turn the chip and soda maker into a healthier business. He served as chief health officer at Vitality, a health and wellness company, and on the Clinton Global Initiative, before making his latest and most controversial move: In 2017, Yach launched the Foundation for a Smoke-Free World, funded by Philip Morris International. Its aim is to reduce tobacco deaths by eliminating combustible tobacco worldwide.

Yach has authored or co-authored over 200 articles on global health in medical journals. Born in South Africa, he is an avid long-distance swimmer and lives in Connecticut, USA.